KT-583-343

MILADY
SalonOvations'

The Multicultural Client: Cuts, Styles, and Chemical Services

LIBRARY
RUGBY COLLEGE

WITHDRAWN

RUGBY COLLEGE of F.E.

* 0 0 6 2 7 6 6 6 *

LIBRARY
RUGBY COLLEGE

Delmar Publishers' Online Services

To access Delmar on the World Wide Web, point your browser to: **http://www.delmar.com/delmar.html**
To access through Gopher: **gopher://gopher.delmar.com**
(Delmar Online is part of "thomson.com", an Internet site with information on more than 30 publishers
of the International Thomson Publishing organization.)
For information on our products and services:
email: info@delmar.com   or   call 800-347-7707

MILADY

SalonOvations'

The Multicultural Client:
Cuts, Styles,
and Chemical Services

Compiled and Written by Victoria Wurdinger

LIBRARY
RUGBY COLLEGE

Milady Publishing Company
(a division of Delmar Publishers)
3 Columbia Circle, Box 12519
Albany, New York 12212-2519

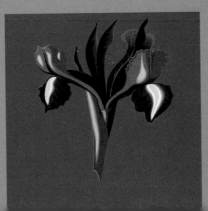

NOTICE TO THE READER

Publisher does not warrant or guarantee any of the products described herein or perform any independent analysis in connection with any of the product information contained herein. Publisher does not assume, and expressly disclaims, any obligation to obtain and include information other than that provided to it by the manufacturer.

The reader is expressly warned to consider and adopt all safety precautions that might be indicated by the activities herein and to avoid all potential hazards. By following the instructions contained herein, the reader willingly assumes all risks in connections with such instructions.

The publisher makes no representation or warranties of any kind, including but not limited to, the warranties of fitness for particular purpose or merchantability, nor are any such representations implied with respect to the material set forth herein, and the publisher takes no responsibility with respect to such material. The publisher shall not be liable for any special, consequential, or exemplary damages resulting, in whole or part, from the readers' use of, or reliance upon, this material.

Cover Design: Susan Mathews/D. Dupras
Cover Photo: Image by Aveda
Illustrations: Shizuko Horii

Milady Staff
Publisher: Catherine Frangie
Acquisitions Editor: Joseph Miranda
Project Editor: Annette Downs Danaher
Production Manager: Brian Yacur

COPYRIGHT © 1996
Milady Publishing Company
(a division of Delmar Publishers)

Printed in the United States of America
Printed and distributed simultaneously in Canada

For more information, contact:
SalonOvations
Milady Publishing Company
3 Columbia Circle , Box 12519
Albany, New York 12212-2519

LIBRARY
RUGBY COLLEGE

ACCESS No. 6276666

CLASS 646.7242

DATE 2 3 MAR 1999

All rights reserved. No part of this work covered by the copyright hereon may be reproduced or used in any form or by any means—graphic, electronic, or mechanical, including photocopying, recording, taping, or information storage and retrieval systems—without the written permission of the publisher.

1 2 3 4 5 6 7 8 9 10   XXX   01 00 99 98 97 96

Library of Congress Cataloging-in-Publication Data

Wurdinger, Victoria.
    SalonOvations' the multicultural client: cuts, styles,
    and chemical services / compiled and written by Victoria Wurdinger.
      p. cm.
    ISBN: 1-56253-178-6
    1. Hairdressing-United States.   2. Hairdressing of Afro-Americans   3. Hispanic Americans-Sevices for.
    4. Asian Americans-Services for.   I. SalonOvation (Firm) II. Title
TT958.W87 1995
646.7'242'089–dc20   95-9955
                                                                 CIP

LIBRARY
RUGBY COLLEGE

CREDITS

Photographer: Preston Phillips

Finished style of a woman wearing a wig
Ariah Perez (model)
Diane Bailey (stylist)
Romell Duresseau (makeup artist)
Photographed on location at Tendrils, Brooklyn, N.Y.

The Halle Berry cut
Andrea Moore (model)
Diane Bailey (stylist)
Romell Duresseau (makeup artist)
Photographed on location at Tendrils, Brooklyn, N.Y.

Short Afro cut
Gregg (model)
Denise "Naeemah" Jeff (stylist)
Romell Duresseau (makeup artist)
Photographed on location at Locks 'N Chops Natural
Hair Salon, New York, N.Y. (Adémola Mandella and
Orin "Nguzi" Saunders, owners)

The Clipper cut
CJ (model)
Denise "Naeemah" Jeff (stylist)
Photographed on location at Locks 'N Chops Natural
Hair Salon, New York, N.Y. (Adémola Mandella and
Orin "Nguzi" Saunders, owners)

The Close Fade
James Davis (model)
Denise "Naeemah" Jeff (stylist)
Photographed on location at Locks 'N Chops Natural
Hair Salon, New York, N.Y. (Adémola Mandella and
Orin "Nguzi" Saunders, owners)

The Wedge
CJ (model)
Denise "Naeemah" Jeff (stylist)
Photographed on location at Locks 'N Chops Natural
Hair Salon, New York, N.Y. (Adémola Mandella and
Orin "Nguzi" Saunders, owners)

The Pompadour
Michael L. Odom (model)
Diane Bailey (stylist)
Photographed on location at Tendrils, Brooklyn, N.Y.

The Wrap
Adrienne Cottrell (model)

Diane Bailey (stylist)
Romell Duresseau (makeup artist)
Photographed on location at Tendrils, Brooklyn, N.Y.

The French Twist
Ariah Perez (model)
Diane Bailey (stylist)
Romell Duresseau (makeup artist)
Photographed on location at Tendrils, Brooklyn, N.Y.

Virgin Relaxer Service
Michael L. Odom (model)
Diane Bailey (stylist)
Photographed on location at Tendrils, Brooklyn, N.Y.

Adhesive Bond Method
Ariah Perez (model)
Diane Bailey (stylist)
Romell Duresseau (makeup artist)
Photographed on location at Tendrils, Brooklyn, N.Y.

Braid and Sew
Kirl Alexander (model)
Diane Bailey (stylist)
Romell Duresseau (makeup artist)
Photographed on location at Tendrils, Brooklyn, N.Y.

Three Strand Cornrowing
Jacqueline Denny (model)
Tulani Kinard (stylist)
Princess Jenkins (makeup artist)
Tina Thomas, Diva Creations (accessories)

Senegalese Twist
Awa Sane (model)
Kirl Alexander (stylist)
Princess Jenkins (makeup artist)
Tina Thomas, Diva Creations (accessories)

Goddess Braids
Dapheney Rodriquez (model)
Fatima Bengouye (stylist)
Princess Jenkins (makeup artist)
Tina Thomas, Diva Creations (accessories)

Casama Braids
Vonnetta Morgan (model)
Fanta Kaba (stylist)
Princess Jenkins (makeup artist)
Tina Thomas, Diva Creations (accessories)

Palm Roll
Tonika Outerbridge (model)
Diane Bailey (stylist)

All braids photographed on location at Tendrils, Brooklyn, N.Y.

Highlighting Relaxed Hair
Adrienne Cottrell (model)
Diane Bailey (stylist)
Romell Duresseau (makeup artist)
Photographed on location at Tendrils, Brooklyn, N.Y.

CONTENTS

CHAPTER 4   *Conducting a Successful Analysis-Based Consultation*   53

CHAPTER 5   *Haircutting-Basic Review and Adjustments by Hair Type*   71

ACKNOWLEGMENTS

This book could not have been written without the unselfish sharing of many. Milady Publishing Company gratefully acknowledges the following individuals, who contributed their time, knowledge, writings and life experience.

Diane Bailey—International Braiders Network, Brooklyn, N.Y.

Tom Brigliadoro—Fantasia, Paramus, N.J.

Robert Brown—Northeast Beauty College, Westland, Mich.

Susan Calandro—Maximus Salon, Merrick, N.Y.

Richard Cardone—Richard Cardone Hair Designers and Color Specialists, Pittsburgh, Penn.

Francine Castle—Personal Image, Wilton, Conn.

Lois Christie—Christie & Co, Bayside, N.Y.

James Christopher Chan—The Hair Resort, Las Vegas, Nev.

D. Dellaquila—Maximus Salon, Merrick, N.Y.

Sheila Dillard—Landover, Md., with special thanks for photo research.

Nekhena Evans—New Bein' Enterprises, Brooklyn, N.Y.

Eric Fisher—Eric Fisher Salon, Wichita, Kansas, and Joico International.

Barry Fletcher and Carol Harper—Avant Garde Hair Gallery, Capital Heights, Md.

Balmer Galindez—D'n'B Salon, N.Y., N.Y., with special thanks for Spanish translations.

Charles Gregory—Charles Gregory Salon, Atlanta, Ga.

Rhonda Hicks and Tommy Hicks—Professional Results Inc.; Emages by Hairstation U.S.A, Houston, Tx.

Laura Hillman O'Brien—Heritage of Beauty, Barber Manufacturing Industry, Washington, DC.

Karen Lafferty—Creative Hairdressers, Falls Church, Va.

Kazunori—Momotaro Salon, NY, N.Y.

Laura Little—NuWave Salon, Bronx, N.Y.

Charlotte Jayne—Garland Drake International, Newport Beach, Calif.

Edward Jimenez—Edward Jimenez Salon, Beverly Hills, Calif.

Katherine Jones—The International Braiders Network, Media, Pa.

Vernice Mark—Historian, The Beauty Culturists League, Detroit, Mich.

Don Marsella—Easy Streaks, NuWave Salon, Bronx, N.Y.

Scott Lee—Soft Sheen Company, Chicago, Ill.

Rocky Plateroti and Franco Marino—Artista for Hair, Scarsdale, N.Y.

Annu Prestonia—Khamit Kinks, Brooklyn, N.Y., and Atlanta, Ga.

Kevin E. Roberts—New Bien' Enterprises, Brooklyn, N.Y.

Jon Rogers—The Place for Hair and Face, Los Angeles, Calif.

Daniel Ruidant—Le Hairdesign, Dallas, Tx.

Rhonda Schamberger—Miss Marion Beauty College, Detroit, Mich.

Keiko Shino—Gardland Drake International; Avantage Salon, Tustin, Calif.

Ruth Sinclair—Khamit Kinks, Atlanta, Ga., and Brooklyn, N.Y.

Ali Syed—Avlon Industries, Bedford Park, Ill.

Joyce Williams—Joyce Williams System, Kansas City, Mo.
Rob Willis—Rob Willis Enterprises, Detroit, Mich.
John Young—Educator, Wahl Clipper Corporation, Pensacola, Fl.

Portions of Chapter 2 were produced in cooperation with the Museum of Cosmetology Arts and Sciences, a project of the Cosmetology Advancement Foundation.

Also, special thanks to the following professionals for their expertise and very helpful input while reviewing this manuscript:
Holly Ann Williams-Pena, DesMoines, Iowa
Linda Jean Crawford, Youngstown, Ohio
Ruth D. Black, Huntsville, Alabama

DEDICATION

This book is dedicated in fond memory to Balmer Galindez, without whose tireless help with Spanish translations and introductions in the Latino community, it would not have been complete. His high standard of professionalism and contributions to all communities will be deeply missed.

INTRODUCTION

The accomplished professional can work with hair of all types. Theoretically, cosmetology school has prepared you for this, but in the working world, styles, techniques and clients change rapidly. To stay ahead of the game, you must change with all three.

This book was created not only to help you stay ahead of changes, but to enable you to invent your own styles, develop personalized techniques and attract and retain new clients throughout your career.

The stylist who has the same client base for decades risks suffering economic ups and downs with those clients and becoming artistically stagnant. However, if you can predict new trends, continually offer new techniques and adjust to shifts in the marketplace, even downturns in the national economy will have minimal effect on your business.

Two of the most dramatic changes that will affect salons through the twenty-first century are the aging of the population and its increasing diversity. As seventy-six million baby boomers enter their fifties, they'll put higher demands on your expertise. Since African Americans, Hispanics and Asians represent the most rapidly growing markets, your proficiency in working with all types of hair and your cultural sensitivity are essential for future growth.

The global village in which we all live is an interdependent community with diverse approaches to beauty, but with at least one important commonality: the desire to look and feel attractive. No one can fulfill this need better than a beauty professional.

In the ever-changing world of hairstyles and fashion, you must know how to perform the latest styles—including cuts, colors, relaxing services and special-occasion styles. Various multicultural markets are discussed here, keying you, the stylist, into hairstyle trends and retail opportunities, so that you can know who your clients are before you begin your work. Then, you will be taken step-by-step through advanced cutting techniques for both men and women, chemical services, a variety of hair-extension techniques and intricate braiding steps—all with full-color illustrations and detailed instructions. You will also learn how to conduct effective client consultations, analyzing hair texture, structure, and the effects of previous chemical services, as well as recommending products for at home care and maintenance.

With this book, we hope you'll celebrate your gift, expand its foundation and enjoy the challenges that each client brings. By mastering multicultural approaches to beauty and working with all varieties of hair, you'll increase your artistic expression, add excitement to your profession and secure your future in the global marketplace.

—Victoria Wurdinger

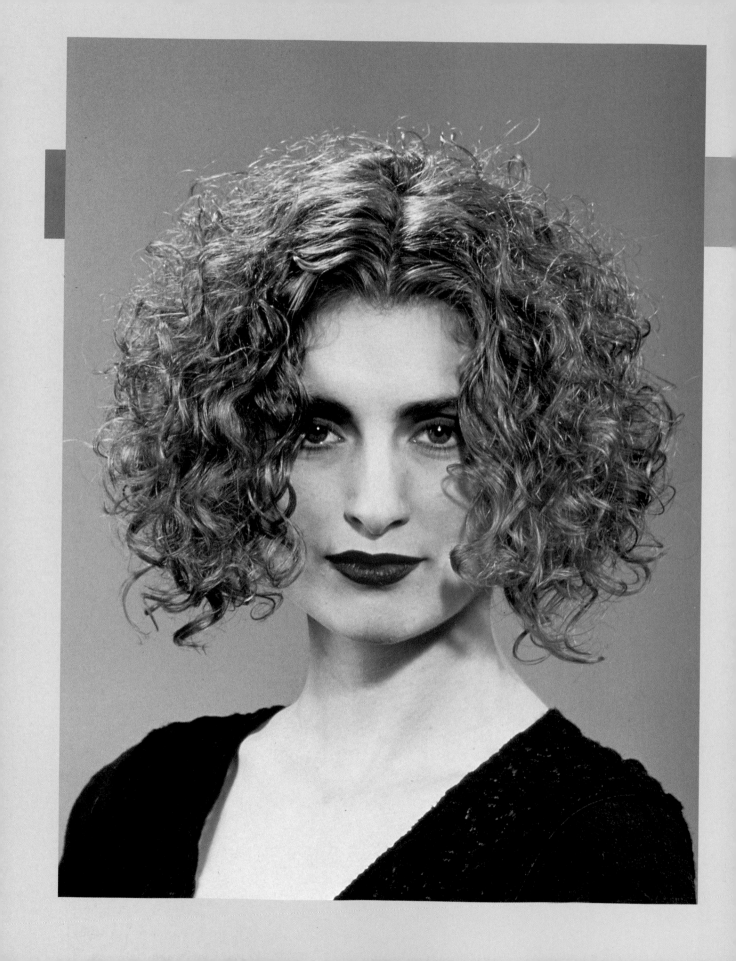

Multicultural Markets

The successful hairdresser of the future will need an expanded repertoire of skills to meet the challenge of America's diverse and brilliant mix of beauty. While once the U.S. was called a melting pot, today it's a bouillabaisse, in which members of many racial, ethnic and cultural groups are celebrating their separate identities. The effects on beauty services are manifold.

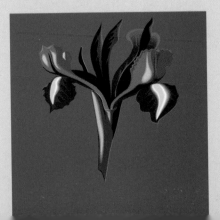

In the early 1970s, the workplace had an imposed one-size-fits-all style that supposedly put employees on the fast-track to success. Today, African braids, Native American ornamentation, shaved heads, and dramatic haircolors and styles that either play up the hair's natural texture or rearrange it entirely are common. For the professional stylist, it's never been a more exciting, creative or challenging time.

To build a clientele, you must be skilled at working with all hair types, textures and densities—and understand the market for your services. That market is more diverse than ever before and it's unlikely that it will ever be considered homogeneous again.

In 1990 the makeup of the U.S. population was:

◆ 76 percent Anglo
◆ 12 percent African American
◆ 9 percent Latino
◆ 3 percent Asian

By 2050 the U.S. Census Bureau projects that the new percentages will be:

◆ 52 percent Anglo
◆ 16 percent African American
◆ 22 percent Latino
◆ 10 percent Asian

America has a new face, and because of it, your success as a stylist depends on more than on a broad range of technical abilities. To truly succeed in an ever-changing marketplace, you'll have to become adept at working with clients whose attitudes toward beauty and its role in their lives differ vastly. The more you are able to overcome cultural differences, the better you'll communicate during a consultation, arrive at the best style solution for the client and deliver it with success.

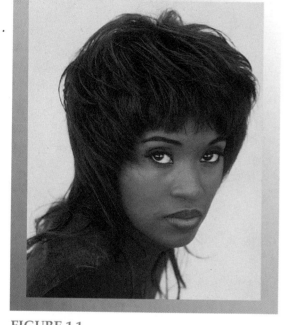

FIGURE 1.1
African-American style. The shag. Hair: Joico International USA Team; Photo: Guillaume Garriague.

POPULATION CHANGES

U. S. Census Bureau demographers, who crunch numbers to determine changes in the population, now group the population into five primary groups: African Americans, Caucasians, Hispanics, Asians and Native Americans. This simplified system of looking at the population's makeup is useful to market researchers, but less pertinent to hairstylists, who must analyze all hair by its type and texture. Hair types from straight and fine to super-curly and extremely dense are found in all segments of the population. However, an overview of demographic changes gives you a colorful picture of the market in which you'll be building a business.

While those who make population predictions also make many assumptions, it's certain that well before the year 2050 the nation's diversity will become extremely evident. Most demographers say that by the year 2010, thirty-nine million Hispanics will represent the largest minority group in the U.S. In certain cities, African Americans will become the dominant population; in others, foreign-born people will represent more than half the population. The latter has already occurred. According to *Newsweek*, Miami's population is 60 percent foreign born; Union City, N.J., has a population that's 55 percent foreign born, and 52 percent of the residents of Monterey Park, Calif., are foreign born.

When it comes to the current crop of young, potential clients, the nation's growing diversity is apparent. The group known as "Generation X" (those born between 1961 and 1981) is comprised of 14 percent African Americans, while the overall population is 12 percent African American. Hispanics represent 12 percent of Generation X versus 9.5 percent of the current total population; Asians are 4 percent of Generation X versus 3 percent of the total population. In San Francisco, 19 percent of the population under eighteen years of age is foreign born.

MARKET CHANGES

The shift in the makeup of the population is just one of the top three changes affecting the ways that services are sold, products are created and businesses are developed. The other two are the aging of the population (the "graying of America") and growing economic disparity, which is creating a two-tiered market. (According to a study by the Census Bureau, in 1992 income for the wealthiest Americans rose by $3,572, but the ranks of the poor grew for the third year in a row.)

CULTURAL DIFFERENCES

A look at each primary market, as delineated by the U.S. Census Bureau, should serve as a guide to building your clientele and as a primer for avoiding the pitfalls experienced by big businesses. For example, when the "Nova" automobile was introduced in Mexico it failed because "no va" means "no go" in Spanish. Another company offered green baseball caps as premiums during a Chinese New Year celebration, unaware that among older generations of Chinese men, wearing a green cap is an announcement that your wife is cheating on you and you want to bring her public scorn. These experiences are particularly important to keep in mind if you want to become a salon owner or independent contractor.

While cultural awareness could save you a caning in Singapore, closer to home it's used by hairstylists who send New Year's greeting cards to clients rather than Christmas cards, which could offend Jewish or Moslem clients; who realize that in some Hispanic cultures women want their husband's approval before dramatically changing their appearance; who recognize that in some other cultures (for example, Orthodox Judaism), touching between men and women is considered sexual, not friendly; and who are aware that for some, lack of eye contact is considered a sign of respect, not an indication that your client isn't listening to you. You'll also learn that women of the Orthodox Jewish and Islamic or Muslim faiths will not be serviced by male cosmetologists or even unveil their hair or remove their wigs in a salon that is occupied by men other than their husbands.

The following information on multicultural markets gives you an overview of each of the most rapidly growing groups, their approach to salon services and what's known about their beauty product and service purchases. While the data was obtained from top researchers and salon-industry professionals, you will always find geographic and individual differences. Let your sensitivity and power of observation be your guide.

AFRICAN AMERICANS

According to the 1990 census, the African-American population is growing twice as fast as the Caucasian population. Between 1980 and 1990, the number of blacks grew by 13.2 percent, while the number of whites increased by 6 percent. Additionally:

◆ The World Almanac reported that thirty million blacks lived in the U.S. in 1990.
◆ The American Health and Beauty Aids Institute (AHBAI) places the African-American population at thirty-one million and projects an increase to thirty-nine million by the year 2021.
◆ According to *American Demographics* magazine, almost one American in eight is black, and in twenty years that proportion will increase to almost one in seven.
◆ Eighty-four percent of African Americans live in urban areas; over 50 percent live in the south.

Salon Spending

It's estimated that African-American women visit a salon once every two weeks, while Caucasian or Anglo women visit salons once every seven weeks. According to Rhonda Hicks of Professional Results, Inc., Houston, Texas, an estimated 35,000 salons in the U.S. specifically service African Americans, who spend and spend an average of fifty dollars per visit. Eighty percent of the spending in these salons is done by women; men account for 10 percent to 20 percent of service and product sales.

Meeting the needs of this client means honing your skills in a number of specific services. According to Hicks, about 96 percent of salons that cater to African Americans provide shampoo and set services, 97 percent offer relaxers, 96 percent offer haircolor and 91 percent perform cutting services. Additionally, 93 percent offer waves and curls, 84 percent offer pressing, 66 percent offer weaving and a growing 39 percent offer braiding.

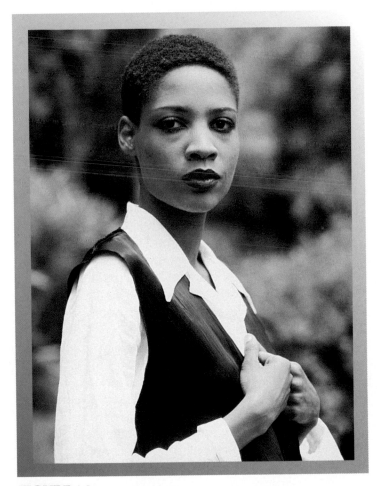

If you want to build your multicultural clientele, these are the areas in which you'll need to be most accomplished. As you develop your expertise in services such as relaxing, you'll discover that your proficiency opens doors to many other markets. Clients who come from the Middle East frequently have abundant, tight curl; Hispanics and Europeans also sometimes request relaxing services.

When it comes to beauty products, all non-Caucasian spending is growing at a rate of 3 percent to 5 percent a year. This rate of growth is faster than that of the salon hair-care market. According to Nancy Flinn Marketing Resources in Weston, Connecticut, professional or salon hair-care sales grew by 2 percent to 3 percent in 1993.

African Americans outspend Caucasians three to one on the beauty-product dollar; 37 percent of all hair-care products ar purchased by blacks, and in 1991 black consumers spent an estimated 600 million dollars on consmetics at all outlets.

African Americans' high rate of spending on beauty products and services is expected to increase even further in the near future, as their earning and

FIGURE 1.2
African-American style. The short afro. Hair: Joico International USA Team;, Photo: Guillaume Garrigue.

spending power increases. Over the last decade, the number of African American households with incomes of 50,000 dollars or more increased by 8 percent, and that rate of increase is expected to accelerate. According to the 1994 *Blackbook* reference guide, black Americans' annual spending power totals 380 billion dollars.

The AHBAI estimates that African Americans spend a total of 1.5 billion dollars a year on professional and mass-market hair-care products. Part of the reason for high spending is that many of the styles worn by this market (for example, relaxers and the two-step perm) require the use of conditioners and maintenance products.

As a salon professional, an important part of your job will be prescribing the correct hair-care products based on hair texture, density, condition, services that have been performed and level of dryness or oiliness. Hairstylists who understand products and their role in total hair care can expect to increase their incomes anywhere from 100 to 1,000 dollars a month, if they possess excellent retailing skills. As spending habits indicate, the African-American market is a highly lucrative one, when it comes to beauty products.

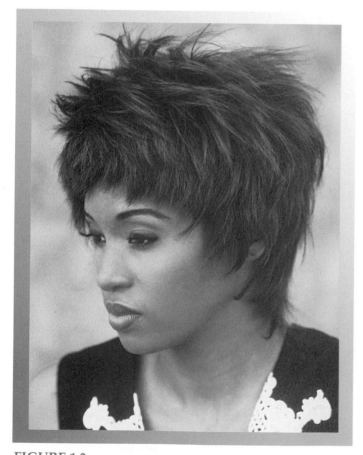

FIGURE 1.3
African-American style. Soft, short layers. Hair: Joico International USA Team; Photo: Guillaume Garrigue.

Hairstyle Trends

Professional hairdressers and product companies alike note that style trends in the African-American market are extremely regional in nature, with the Afrocentric influence strongest in the East, and curls and body waves in vogue in the Southeast. While relaxing is a popular service among all professionals, it is the least popular in the carefree West. Within these broad and generalized geographic ranges are pockets with their own trends. Detroit is known for creative men's cuts; Brooklyn, N.Y., is practically the braiding capital of the U.S.; cities such as New Orleans, which is extremely humid in summer, see more seasonal style changes.

Braiding has become popular among younger clients, who are highly influenced by the styles worn by movie stars and musicians. And since pop icons tend to change their hairstyles frequently, so too will your younger clientele. In this market, what's hot today is not tomorrow.

Currently larger braids are in favor, and ornamentation is extremely popular. Women who get this look can go two to three months without a salon visit, until the braids need adjusting. Social trends also affect which hairstyles are in vogue. Braids and natural styles increased in popularity as pride in heritage evolved into social and political statements, and Europeans were less able to impose their values and sense of style on others.

One relatively new style that also lasts two weeks without a salon visit is "the freeze." Kansas City, Missouri, stylist Joyce Williams is credited with its creation—and its apt name. It uses ample amounts of product, applied to hair that has been previously relaxed or curled. The style is dried and frozen in place; it can then be left as is, molded into finger-

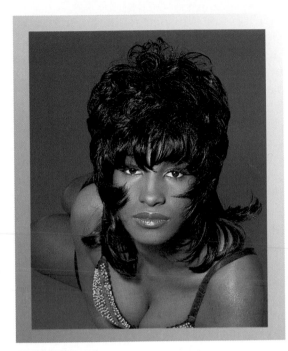

FIGURE 1.4
African-American style. A nouveau shag. Hair: Barbara Marshall and Rhonda Hicks for Professional Results International, Inc. and Emages by Hair Station USA, Houston; Makeup: Mikal; Photo: Josef Berard.

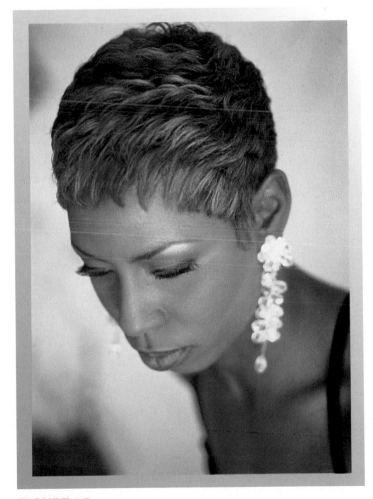

FIGURE 1.5
African-American style. A layered crop. Hair: Barbara Marshall and Rhonda Hicks for Professional Results International, Inc. and Emages by Hair Station USA, Houston; Makeup: Mikal; Photo: Josef Berard.

waves, pulled into a pompadour or finished with an iron and sprayed for extra hold. Eighteen to twenty-five-year-olds, who don't require extremely professional looks, are the biggest market for the style, and you'll learn about it later in Chapter 9. Additionally, the big Afro is making a comeback, although its popularity is definitely regional and possibly short-lived.

The third biggest hairstyle trend involves hair additions. Various types of hair-addition services are equally popular with younger women and those who want to expand the range of their natural hair. With older clients, woven-in wefts of hair can be used to conceal thinning areas. Afrocentric braids are among the most popular additions, and they can be attached in many ways. Hair wefts or extensions and braids can be made of human or synthetic hair. Long wefts of several individual pre-braided strands can be attached just like full weaves; sections of unbraided hair fiber can be attached individually and turned into thick casama braids and Sengalese twists.

Additionally, stylists say that 85 percent of their African-American clients wear haircolor. It is the fastest growing service in many salons. Influence from superstars, such as Whitney Houston and Janet Jackson, has created a renewed interest in haircolor, as have safer haircoloring products, which can be used in conjunction with relaxers and curls.

Men are open to style changes as well, and business styles are more diverse and individual than ever. In general, professional looks are close-cut and partially textured to control the curl pattern, although natural curl is frequently used to advantage. In the Midwest, men are sporting 1950s' pompadours and are partially texturizing or totally straightening their hair; in the East, men are experimenting with a wide variety of looks and shapes.

Marketing to African Americans

As recently as ten years ago, product companies and advertisers all but ignored the African-American market. Today, men and women of color are targeted by many. African Americans are a diverse group with a wide range of skin tones and hair textures that encompass everything from extremely curly to naturally straight. Naturally curly African hair permits an astonishing array of styles that are achieved in myriad ways, presenting a highly creative outlet for the accomplished stylist.

To capture this market, become committed to learning more about it. Start by recognizing that it encompasses a wide range of consumers with clearly different needs from what market researchers call the "mass market." Do not look at this market—or any other for that matter—as being a single, homogeneous unit. It is comprised of people whose roots are as close as the Caribbean, as far away as Australia, third and fourth-generation Americans, Africans and many others, whose cultural values and style preferences vary widely.

In this market, salons generate most of their income from relaxing, coloring and perming. Extension and braiding services are growing quickly. Become more proficient in these services and you're bound to attract a diverse clientele—if you court them. Salons that display posters of all types of models and hairstyles are taking a step in the right direction.

If you advertise your services, advertise in a wide variety of newspapers, including those that target African-American readers. Carry products appropriate for all hair types and needs. Also, do not neglect the importance of community involvement. As a stylist, take part in community events, give away haircuts and salon services at local fund-raisers and make it known that you understand how to work with all types of hair.

According to Larry Glover of the J. Curtis Company in Montclair, New Jersey, keep these points in mind when attempting to capture your share of the African-American Market:

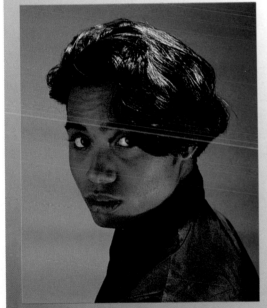

FIGURE 1.6
Hispanic-American style. Hair: Sabrina Hill for John Paul Mitchell Systems.

◆ Status and prestige often influence major purchase decisions.
◆ African Americans are not dark-skinned white people and should not be treated as such in advertising.
◆ African Americans are responsive to marketing attempts, when a personal invitation is extended.
◆ You should have a specific strategy to attract African Americans, because they lead the way in the "browning of America."
◆ Cultural differences require that you understand the people who will be your customer base in the future. Fifty-five percent of African Americans regard ethnicity as more important than nationality.

HISPANIC AMERICANS

The fastest growing market in the U.S. is the Hispanic market.

◆ Between 1980 and 1990, the Hispanic population grew by more than 50 percent, gaining an additional 7.7 million persons.
◆ In 1990, the census counted over 22 million Americans of Hispanic origin.

◆ By the year 2010, there may be 39 million Hispanics in the United States.

Projections for the future Hispanic population are based on birthrates, immigration and other factors. It was previously assumed that U.S. fertility rates would decline through 2050; now it looks as though they will remain constant. After the 1990 census figures were used to create projections, a new 1993 report from the Census Bureau anticipated 500,000 additional immigrants.

One of the changes in the new report is that the Census Bureau, which once projected populations for Caucasians, African Americans and Asians only, has now added projections for American Indians and Hispanics.

New projections for Hispanics of all races show an increase from twenty-four million in 1992 to eighty-one million in 2050. That would result in a staggering increase from 9 percent of the total population to 21 percent of the population. Indeed, Hispanics are expected to account for 57 percent of population growth between the years 2030 and 2050.

While market researchers consider Hispanics to be a specific marketing group that you can target, the Census Bureau treats Hispanics as a group that overlaps racial categories. Four percent of blacks are Hispanic in origin, coming from Puerto Rico, the Dominican Republic and Brazil, among other countries. In twenty Hispanic subgroups, what they have in common is as obvious as what they don't. But despite the incredible diversity among Hispanic Cubans, Mexicans, Puerto Ricans, South Americans and Europeans, market researchers claim that one factor holds true of all: Hispanics are extraordinarily brand loyal when compared to the rest of the population.

For the professional stylist, this means that if you sell the hair-care products that your Hispanic clientele prefers, chances are excellent that they will continue to come to you for that brand. If Hispanics like patronizing your salon for services, they are less likely than other clients to change salons.

Salon Spending

Hispanics as a group have never been part of widely published, salon-specific market research, if at all. (Most research is done on the behalf of major product manufacturers, such as food companies.) However, a survey by Market Segment Research (MSR), Miami, Florida, measured which health and beauty aids African Americans, Hispanics and Asian Americans buy. It revealed that 93 percent of Hispanics buy shampoo (compared to 76 percent of blacks and 89 percent of Asians), 61 percent buy conditioner (compared to 52 percent of blacks and 59 percent of Asians) and 27 percent buy hairspray. The U.S. magazine network claims that Hispanics are the biggest users of health and beauty aids.

While there is no available data showing salon versus mass-market purchases, given the loyalty factor, Hispanics who become accustomed to buying in a salon will probably continue to do so.

Like the African-American market, the Hispanic market has grown in terms of household income. During the last decade, the number of Hispanic families with annual incomes of 50,000 dollars-grew by almost 50 percent. In 1993 their total purchasing power reached 200 billion dollars.

As researchers continue to study the diverse Hispanic market, figures on salon patronization and service expenditures may emerge. To date, what's known remains in the hands of private companies, who paid "quite a few dollars" for the data. One cultural preference that has been noted is that sex segregation is a strong component in beauty salons, as it is in the Asian market. Hispanic men are more likely to patronize a barber shop than a full-service salon. But as Hispanic salons evolve, this, too, will change.

Hairstyle Trends

Market Segment Research's survey revealed that the typical Hispanic consumer lags behind U.S. trends by five years. Health and fitness is not a priority with this market. According to top salon stylists, the current trend among Hispanics is a move from a very stylized look toward softer styles. Perms are extremely popular, and Hispanic women as a group tend to view long hair as more feminine, although there are always exceptions. Currently, haircolor is subtler and warmer than ever before, as Hispanic women discover the range of color selections and application techniques used in salons. However, Hispanic women tend to prefer bolder fashion and makeup colors than other markets do, according to several cosmetic manufacturers.

Hispanic hair types are as diverse as African Americans', if not more so, due to strong subgroups and a racial mix that includes light-skinned and black Hispanics. On the West Coast, Hispanics of South American/Indian origin dominate, and their hair tends to be straighter; on the East Coast, Puerto Ricans, who have curlier hair, represent a large portion of the Hispanic population.

Perming for soft waves, partial relaxing services (or hair texturizing) and haircolor are currently the biggest dollar-producing services in the Hispanic market, according to Hispanic stylists. Perming has long been a mainstay, while haircolor is among the fastest growing services.

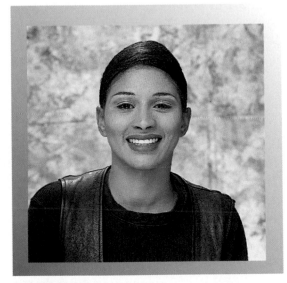

FIGURE 1.7
Hispanic-American style.

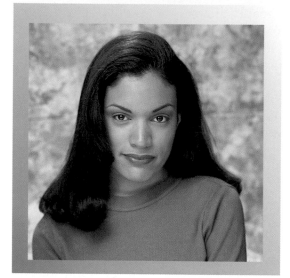

FIGURE 1.8
Hispanic-American style.

Marketing to Hispanics

If you don't speak the language, targeting the Hispanic market naturally becomes more difficult. However, it is by no means impossible for the non-Spanish-speaker.

If you wish to attract Hispanic clients to your chair, examine the subgroup in your geographic area; do not view Hispanics as one homogeneous group. Country of origin, length of U.S. residency and socioeconomic status will determine their attitude toward salons and salon services, not the simple fact that they're Hispanic. Discover the needs of Hispanic women in your area and set out to prove that you can meet them.

Hispanics are concentrated geographically. In 1985 one-third lived in California and nearly 88 percent were concentrated in California, Texas, New York, Florida, Illinois, New Jersey, New Mexico, Arizona and Colorado.

Advertising to this market is more likely to succeed if you do it through the community or through electronic media.

According to Filiberto Fernandez, Senior Vice President of Marketing for the Telemundo Group, Inc., any attempt to capture the Hispanic market must include a heavy measure of community involvement. Knowledge of statistics alone will rarely lead to success.

Hispanic stylists say that making the Hispanic woman feel comfortable in your chair is of utmost importance. Sometimes she will shy away from salons that appear to have "snob appeal." A personalized and caring service attitude will ensure repeat clients.

Keep in mind that Hispanic women are particularly sensitive about their hair-length preferences. Display posters of Hispanic women in current hairstyles and let the Hispanic woman consider a style change over a period of time; don't ever push her into making a quick decision—particularly if a dramatic change is involved. If she is married, ask her if she would like to call her husband to discuss her new look before proceeding with a service.

And, of course, familiarize yourself with a wide variety of hair types and textures. You should know when to use a relaxer and when to use a perm solution to gently texturize a super-curly hairline when the rest of the hair has medium curl. If you find there is a language barrier, communicate in the universal language of photos.

Salon owners would be wise to hire Spanish-speaking stylists; stylists who make an effort to learn the language will find that it opens doors to greater understanding and communication. Given this group's explosive growth, salons and stylists that court them—and make an attempt to understand the diversity of this group—should find there's a bright future ahead.

ASIAN AMERICANS

The number of Asian Americans doubled between 1980 and 1990, growing from 3.7 million to 7.3 million persons. Additionally:

◆ Census Bureau projections show the Asian and Pacific Islander population growing at a rate of 4 percent annually during the 1990s.

◆ By the year 2000, Asian Americans could number more than twelve million.

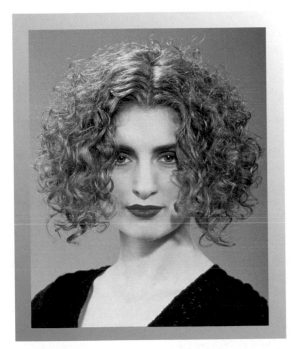

FIGURE 1.9
Asian-American style. Hair: Denice Hanson for John Paul Mitchell Systems; Photo: J.D. Chielli.

The recent Asian population increases were largely due to immigration, primarily among Vietnamese, Koreans, Asian Indians and Filipinos. The largest Asian-American subgroup is Chinese, which in 1990 numbered 1.7 million. Additionally, in 1990 there were 1.4 million Filipinos, 850 thousand Japanese, 815 thousand Asian Indians and 790 million Koreans living in the United States.

Like the Hispanic market, the Asian-American market is comprised of diverse subgroups that have unique cultural attitudes, based on their country of origin. Unlike Hispanics, they do not share a common language, making marketing especially difficult. (China alone has 100 different dialects; there are 90 dialects in the Philippines.) However, Asians are more likely to speak English at home, particularly if they are not foreign-born. Market Segment Research found that, unlike Hispanics, most Asian Americans do not speak their own language exclusively. Just 33 percent do, and a quarter speak both English and their native tongue equally.

While many Caucasians presume that all Asians have thick, straight, black hair, in reality many Asians have curly hair, and black is a matter of what the eye sees. Haircolor professionals say Asian hair is truly dark, dark brown. Their evidence: when it is decolorized, it does go through a red stage; if it were pure black, they say, it wouldn't.

According to hair-care product manufacturers, Asian hair does have its own unique characteristics. These presumed differences—and the debate they create—will be examined later; for now, remember that perming any hair type requires an in-depth understanding of its complex and varying structures.

Asian Americans intermarry with Caucasians more than any other group. According to *Newsweek* magazine, Japanese Americans marry non-Japanese about 65 percent of the time, and, since 1981, the number of children born in the U.S. with one Japanese and one Caucasian parent has exceeded the number with two Japanese parents. Given this, the concept of defining hair as having strictly "Asian characteristics" makes less and less sense. For that matter, intermarriage among all groups continuously blurs the lines which previously defined hair types. The Census Bureau itself (not without controversy) is considering creating new categories that permit respondents to declare themselves by particular mixed backgrounds, displaying their pride in both.

Salon Spending

When it comes to salon spending habits, the least is know about Asian Americans. Marketing service companies have only recently begun to study and target Asian Americans, and their attempts are strewn with classic mistakes.

For instance, it is known that more than any other group, Asians are value shoppers. According to *Promo* magazine, one marketer used this information and decided to issue native-language coupons to Chinese consumers. The coupons offered a twenty-four dollar discount, but in some Chinese communities, the number 2 is close to the word for "easy" and the number 4 is close to the word for "death." The point: Many times, native-language advertising campaigns get lost in translation.

One available statistic on beauty spending indicates that Asian Americans purchase more hairspray than African Americans or Hispanics. According to MSR, 89 percent of Asians purchase shampoo and 59 percent purchase conditioners.

Salons that specifically target Asians have existed as long as Asian neighborhoods have; in New York's Chinatown there are more than ten within a two-block area. Salons in Asian communities are generally staffed by native-language speakers and offer a range of hair services, but frequently fall short of having a complete, full-service menu. In the U.S., Asian salons and the attitude toward them is likely to mirror the attitudes of their owners' and patrons' country of origin.

For many Asians, salon visits were an expensive and sometimes unattainable luxury in their country of origin. The obvious exception is Japan, which in 1992 had 187,000 salons, employing 315 thousand hairdressers, and 144 thousand barber shops, employing 240 thousand barbers. In Japan and many other Asian countries, beauty care is segregated by sex.

Second-, third- and fourth-generation Asians are likely to patronize a mainstream salon they trust; according to one Japanese stylist, the primary thing to keep in mind is that classically dense, coarse Asian hair shows a cutting mistake much more easily than European hair does. The biggest perming mistake stylists tend to make with Asian clients is over-processing the hair.

Hairstyle Trends

Given the diversity of the Asian market, pinpointing style trends becomes a study in country of origin, length of time in the U.S. and generational differences. For example, in Japan younger women prefer perms and revert to natural-textured looks as they grow older; in the U.S. the opposite is more often true. Young, stylish Japanese favor long hair, bobs and fashionable, geometric cuts. Perms are popular among Chinese women over thirty.

According to *Face*, a California-based publication aimed at all Asian women, in general recent immigrants prefer perms over coloring, and Asian Americans who have been in the U.S. for an extended period of time prefer coloring over perms—particularly if they are in their 20s.

Numerous Asian clients get haircolor, which is a surprise to many Caucasians. In Japan the salon haircoloring business increased in percentage of gross by 15.6 percent between 1990 and 1991. However, haircolor is most frequently used as a style statement. Asians, like Native Americans, East Indians, Native Alaskans and many others, are less likely to experience a preponderance of gray hair than those of European ancestry.

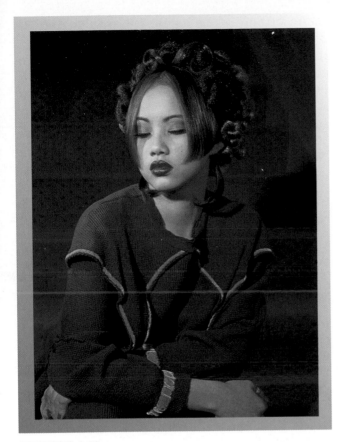

FIGURE 1.10
Asian-American style. Hair: Philip Pelusi International Design Team; Makeup: Valerie Gatchell; Photo: Philip Pelusi.

Marketing to Asian Americans

According to the Asia Link Consulting Group in New York, more than half the Asian population in the U.S. lives in Los Angeles, San Francisco, New York, Honolulu and Chicago. Their average household income, $38,450, is higher than the U.S. average.

Market Segment Research's survey notes that Asians are more likely to shop by price than African Americans or Hispanics, and they are as likely to buy a sale item as they are a familiar brand. Japanese Americans are the most likely to pay higher prices for quality beauty products, according to cosmetic manufacturers.

While marketers emphasize that Asian Americans tend to be value shoppers, this does not necessarily mean that you can lure them with promotions. According to one Japanese executive quoted in *Promo* magazine, Japanese are not familiar with coupons and perceive their use as shameful.

As with all other markets, targeting them means becoming involved in the community at all levels. Asia Link Consulting Group notes that community involvement and word-of-mouth advertising will bring the most success; advertising is also effective.

Advertise in newspapers that can prove they have a significant number of Asian -readers and position your skills as applicable to all clients and all hair types. While much of target marketing is up to the salon owner, individual stylists can do many things to attract a diverse clientele, beginning with a diverse education.

ATTRACTING MULTICULTURAL CLIENTS

New stylists have a choice of salons in which to work and frequently base their decisions on the clientele a salon attracts. When you interview at a salon, notice whether the salon services older, upscale clients or a young, highly fashionable crowd. If it is not attracting a multicultural clientele, ask the owner about increasing the salon's market share and let him or her know that you are educated in working with all hair types.

Develop a plan for attracting a range of clients in conjunction with the owner, who controls the advertising budget. If you intend to work as an independent contractor, advertising is in your hands and you'd be wise to spend about 5 percent of your annual income to attract new clients.

Other ways of attracting a wide range of clientele that have proven successful include:

◆ Send press releases to local newspapers, TV and radio stations announcing that you have recently joined a salon and are skilled at working with all types of hair. Don't be afraid to promote yourself.

◆ Offer to do makeovers for local cable TV stations and newspaper beauty columns. Get a group of talented artists together and pay a professional photographer to photograph models you've made over. Include models from all backgrounds and cultures and send the photos to local beauty editors.

◆ Approach local organizations, particularly multicultural ones, and let them know that you're willing to donate your services during fund-raisers. Offer to do makeover's for their board members or at least style their hair for public appearances. Word of mouth works!

◆ If local regulations permit, set up a chair at street fairs and do haircuts for everyone to see, at a discounted price. Or donate what you make to a community group that serves your target market. Find out more about the market through your relationship with them.

◆ Find clients who you can style or make over and take snapshots of the person both before your services and in your finished style. Display them at your station.

◆ If you want to build business, don't leave it all up to the salon owner. Go to banks, local department stores and other businesses in your area and approach employees who are highly visible with an offer they can't refuse. Cut or style their hair for free, in return for referrals, should anyone ask who did their hair. Give them your business card to hand out. When you do this, target clients from all backgrounds and cultures.

◆ If you are a salon owner or plan to be one, try these ideas. Involve your entire salon in the effort to target clients from all walks of life. Hold styling nights or fashion shows in the salon in conjunction with other businesses that already attract the clients you've targeted. Hiring a multicultural staff is one of the quickest ways to tell the community that you service all its members.

◆ As an owner, frequently update your staff's education, display several different magazines that are aimed at specific groups and both sexes in your reception area and update your salon posters frequently. Carefully select the product lines you carry, including hair-care lines aimed at Hispanic, Asian and African Americans and makeup lines for women of color. In other words, carry your multicultural message throughout your entire salon.

◆ Remember that local dance clubs often attract young clients from all walks of life. Patronize them, not only to observe the styles that are in vogue, but offer makeover's to their staff, network and pass out your business card or even take part in an event. Such clubs often hold fashion shows, for which you can style the hair. This not only nets you business and spreads your reputation as a multicultural stylist, it helps you do something else that is vital to multicultural marketing. It keeps you on top of the trends.

◆ Adjust the hours you work to accommodate the clientele you want to attract. Add magazines in your waiting room that are of special interest to multicultural clients; use posters and window signs that target a wide range of clients.

Non-Caucasian "minorities" now make up 25 percent of the U.S. population, but by the year 2010 non-Caucasians will comprise one-third of the total population. By the year 2040 they will represent more than 40 percent of the population. Total consumer spending among these groups is currently more than 600 billion dollars; this figure will grow as their ranks do.

Growing your business for the future means meeting the needs of a diverse America. But, diversity is not new. Many hold that the U.S. was never a "melting pot," but a place where segments of the population always maintained separate cultural identities. If your multicultural business can help them do that—and underscore the pride in all types of beauty—you've build a strong foundation for the future.

STAYING AHEAD OF THE TRENDS

Successful stylists not only keep on top of style trends, they stay ahead of them. How do they do it? By knowing from where trends originate. If you read only mainstream magazines, you're barely keeping up with trends, after the fact.

Music videos are among the first places to look. Often trends originate on the streets and show up first on networks such as MTV. Pay attention to the Paris collections, which borrow liberally from street trends all over the world. Stay on top of the youth market as much as you do the professional market, regardless of your current clientele. It'll make your career much more creative and exciting and prevent you from getting into a rut!

Take part in advanced education as often as possible. Attend trade shows aimed at various markets—not just the big, mainstream ones—and sign up for a class. Even if you subscribe to only a few magazines, regularly skim others at the magazine rack. You don't have to buy them all; find a newsstand that isn't hostile to browsers. Look at magazines that are specifically aimed at the African-American, Hispanic and Asian markets, noting not only which topics they cover, but the hairstyles portrayed on the cover, in their advertising and in fashion and beauty features.

If you travel for fun or business, drop by salons in the area, introduce yourself and ask a few questions about regional trends or specific techniques used in the salon. Tell the receptionist that you are a stylist and that you are interested in by what you saw, walking by. Most will be happy to chat with you. Then invite the owner or stylists to visit your salon, if they're ever in your area. At home, visit neighborhoods other than your own and observe what you see on the streets and in the windows of salons. (It's a great way to compare pricing, too!)

Keep your eye on fashion centers such as London, Paris and Madrid, which frequently set trends years before they come to the U.S. Mixing up styles, multiculturally speaking, appeared on the streets of London years ago, where Asians and Anglos were seen sporting African locks, and East Indians change their natural hair texture with perms.

While some clients prefer styles that underscore pride in their heritage, others enjoy adapting what works best for them at the moment. In a world of fashion choices, understanding hair in all its diverse ranges gives you skills that are bound only by an individual's personal sense of style. In instances where that sense of style is culturally oriented, the more you know about various markets, local communities and cultural attitudes, the better off you'll be.

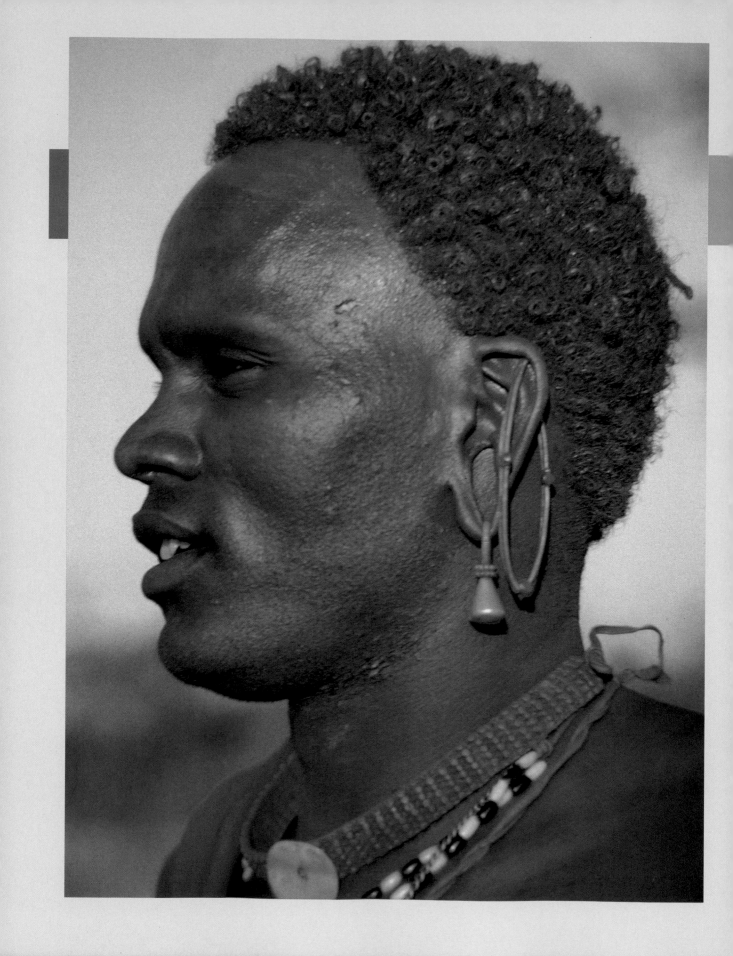

Roots – Locks 'Round the Clock

To paraphrase Milton, beauty is nature's way of bragging. And while nature has bragged throughout history in myriad ways, hairstylists have always helped her flaunt her stuff. Many of today's styles can be traced back to traditional styles, dating back thousands of years.

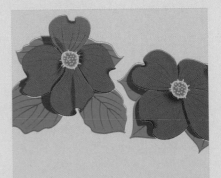

According to a French historian, the first haircut was done by draping hair across a rock and using a stone to hack it off. The effect must have looked worse than a cut done with pinking shears, although beauty is always in the eye of the beholder. It could be considered the first textured style or shag. At any rate, flaked stone tools, which could have been used for cutting, date back to the Middle Paleolithic period, from 100,000 B.C. to 35,000 B.C.

AFRICAN INNOVATIONS

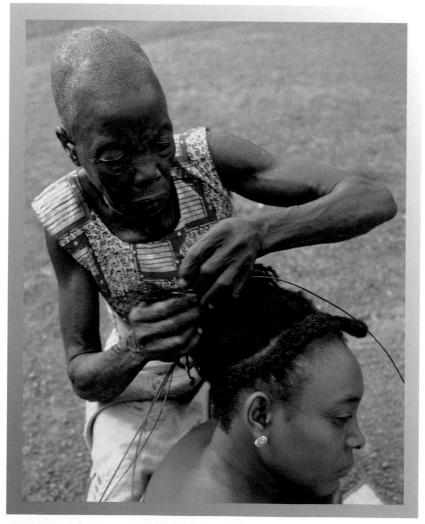

FIGURE 2.1
Mangbetu chief's principal wife having hair styled in traditional manner. Photo: Eliot Elisofon, 1970; National Museum of African Art, Eliot Elisofon Photographic Archives, Smithsonian Institution.

The first highly decorative hairstyles were noted among African tribes, which used hair to make important social and cultural statements. Often, specific styles of braiding indicated whether a woman was single, in mourning, was celebrating the birth of her first child or was of high social rank. In some tribes, hair length was a measure of strength; in others, cutting the hair was a way of driving out evil spirits, which were thought to enter the body through the hair.

Many tribes were and still are identified by their distinctive hairstyles. Women of the Masai tribe of Kenya wind their hair into an elaborate bob. The Zulus set highly unusual styles in place with the aid of mud. Many other tribes still create twisted ringlets, plaits and locks, using various types and colors of clay.

Throughout history, asymmetrical cuts were used to indicate age or profession. The royal runners of the Dahomey Empire shaved one side of the head and carefully shaped the opposite into a fuller style. In Egypt, barbers created a "Horus lock," which was a long lock left to fall over one ear that signified youth.

ANCIENT EGYPTIAN STYLES

Hairstyles—and the cosmetology profession—were well documented by scribes of ancient Egypt. For almost 3,000 years, style changes in Egypt were minimal. The women of Egypt wore extremely elaborate plaiting, which was decorated with shells, sequins and glass or gold beads. Particular styles were a sign of social status, and the average citizen would never wear the same style as the queen, unless she was prepared to lose it, along with her head. Between 3000 and 1596 B.C., the Egyptians moved from wearing braided styles to favoring wigs. Men invariably shaved their heads and wore wigs; women cut their hair very short and wore wigs made of human hair or sheep's wool, because it was closest to their natural texture. Flax or palm-fibre were also used to create wigs, and examples were found in early tombs.

The cosmetology trade had its own hierarchy in Egypt. Barbers for the wealthy visited clients in their homes each morning and attended to their styling needs, as well as to their nails. It is notable that barbers were sometimes doctors, a tradition that continued well into the tenth century, when French barber-surgeons joined to form their own organization. Traveling barbers, who were primarily patronized by the poor, sat under trees waiting for passers-by to become clients. Anointing the hair with essential oils, such as Sandalwood and Frankenscense, was an important part of dressing locks.

Egyptians were clean-shaven or wore fake, decorated beards, but the first formal record of shaving is found among the Romans in the fourth century B.C. Alexander the Great is credited with introducing the trend; supposedly he was afraid that during hand-to-hand combat, his men could be seized by their beards. Later beards became a sign of high social position, until the Emperor Constantine brought back shaving, around the fourth century A.D.

Henna was used to color hair—as were berry juices. Both also served as cosmetics. Indeed, an excellent argument could be made that ancient Egypt was the birth place of the true art of cosmetology. It is also said that Egyptian women bathed in sour milk; milk is a source of alpha hydroxy acids, which are much touted in skin care today.

The women of Morocco and the Middle East also used henna, in a highly unique fashion. In what may be the first form of tattooing, women created elaborate and stunningly beautiful designs using various shades of henna, which stained the skin and nails. Frequently this ancient art was part of a marriage ritual, and it can still be seen today.

ARCHAEOLOGICAL EVIDENCE

Throughout the world, ancient paintings and scrolls show that hairstyles were almost always a measure of social status. Painted ceilings in palaces on the island of Crete provide further insight into the ancient art of hairdressing. The Cretans, who lived around 2000 B.C. to 1400 B.C., had thick, dark hair that was either naturally curly or artificially curled and waved. Many ancient peoples were familiar with oils, waxes and unguents, and the Cretans used them to set their hair into structured waves and curls. More elaborate hairstyles were worn at the court; the poor wore simplified versions of those styles. Waxes and oils were also used in ancient Persia to create curls.

In India, which boasts one of the oldest civilizations in the world, oral tradition took precedence over writing until about 1200 B.C. but ancient paintings can be seen that depict women in long, heavy braids.

Perhaps the oldest hairstyle that was not a wig ever seen firsthand by archaeologists is braids, which were noted on mummies found in China. The mummies were astonishingly well-preserved, because they were found in the northwest foothills and the fringes of the Taklimakan Desert, where daytime temperatures soar above 100 degrees.

While Egyptian mummies are older, few retained their real hair, and they were often found wearing wigs. The Chinese mummies were an important find, because they appeared almost exactly as the people did in real life.

Surprisingly, they were not of Chinese descent, but were blonde and light-brown-haired Caucasians, who could have traveled from Europe or the Ukraine. All the women wore several long braids, and a child wore a tattoo on her wrist. Resting with them were wooden combs. However, these relatively simple braids were nothing like the astonishing works of art found in early African civilizations.

Heated tools were used to style hair as early as the fifth or fourth century B.C. A glazed brick relief piece of art, which is displayed at the Louvre in Paris today, depicts Susa warriors from Iran (Persia) with curly hair and beards. Historians surmise that the perfectly shaped curls were created with hot tongs, probably heated over a flame.

HAIRCOLOR HISTORY

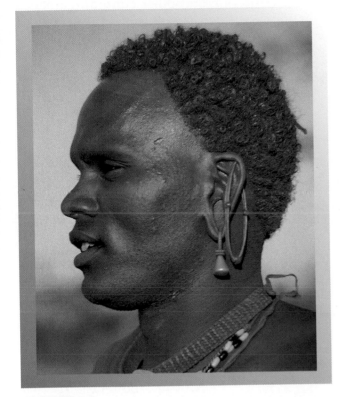

FIGURE 2.2
Hair and body art. Maasai junior elder, Manyara, Tanzania.
Photo: Eliot Elisofon, 1966; National Museum of African Art,
Eliot Elisofon Photographic Archives, Smithsonian Institution.

Haircolor has its own colorful history. African tribes used red ochre and animal fat to color their hair; some say that one of the earliest formulas for covering gray hair was an African one that used bull's blood cooked in oil.

It is believed that in 27 B.C., the Gauls dyed their hair red to indicate class rank. At this time there were no natural redheads in existence, at least that were ever depicted or documented.

The first documented natural redhead appeared in Scotland during the Dark Ages. Scientists believe that it was a genetic mistake. Because of red's surprising appearance—and its unfortunate timing—the haircolor became associated with witchcraft.

Blonde, on the other hand, was noted much earlier in history. How did blondes get their reputation for having more fun? Roman law decreed that yellow or blonde was to be worn by "women of the night." Later, during the Renaissance, women favored golden hues and considered them angelic. They enhanced blonde shades by mixing black sulfur, alum and honey, applying it to their hair and spreading their tresses over a brimless hat until the sun helped them achieve the desired shade. Centuries later, Hollywood restored blondes' reputation as the bad girls of society, or at least as its sex symbols.

AFTER THE YEAR ZERO

The Anastazi, who lived in prehistoric times and developed basket-making and agricultural techniques as early as 100 A.D.; are now extinct, although the adobe houses they lived in around 700 A.D. can still be seen in the Southwest. Evidence shows that they, too, favored braids. After the Anastazi disappeared, certain Native American tribes shaved their hair into fierce-looking Mohawks, imitated in recent times by punk rockers. Many used feathers in elaborate head-dresses or to adorn simple styles.

Like many groups, Native Americans discovered that the way they wore their hair, which emphasized cultural pride, caused strong reactions in Europeans. Hair became something to fear, both because it was different and because it was seen as a refusal to give up the past, or assimilate. As any student of history knows, the easiest way to suppress a population is to deny them their history and their culture.

The wearing of Native-American and other cultural hairstyles brought about discriminatory acts, such as expulsion from school, as recently as the early 1970s; African-American women were dismissed from jobs around the same time for wearing traditional African braids. The Afro became a political statement, which also brought about strong reactions. In 1967 a member of the Afro American Students Union at the University of California told a white reporter from the *New York Times*, "We decided to stop hating ourselves, trying to look like you...straightening our hair."

According to the *Encyclopedia of Pop Culture*, the Afro lost favor when non-blacks began wearing it. Art Garfunkel's hair was called an "Isro" (a reference to his Jewish/Israeli heritage), and non-Jewish whites who wore their hair full and curly called the style an "Anglo." Interestingly, the *Encyclopedia of Pop Culture* also notes that in the 1970s, the government of Tanzania in Africa outlawed Afros because they had become an "emblem of western cultural colonialism, favored by fashion-conscious members of Tanzania's decadent elite."

Even today, African Americans who embrace the ancient tradition of hairlocking and proudly wear a style that has been often called "Dreadlocks," and is now respected as "African Locks," are discovering that discrimination in employment is still a real and present threat.

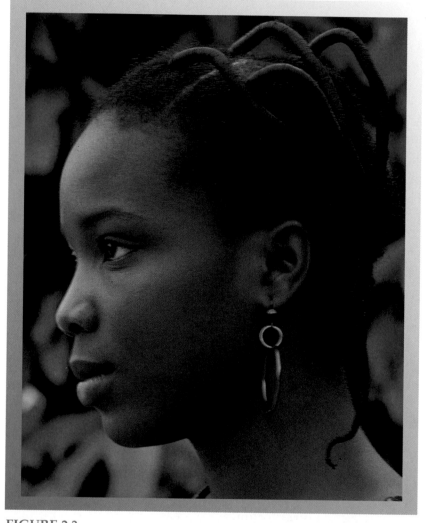

FIGURE 2.3
Yoruba girl with hair wrapped in black thread, Nigeria. Photo: Eliot Elisofon, 1970; National Museum of African Art, Eliot Elisofon Photographic Archives, Smithsonian Institution.

But the suppression, acceptance and frequent mainstream adaptation of various cultural hairstyles occurred over hundreds of years. During that time, African Americans in particular adapted unique ways of dealing with the situation. The techniques they developed are used by every cosmetologist today to style curly hair.

EARLY DEVELOPMENT OF MODERN AMERICAN HAIRSTYLES AND TECHNIQUES

When African slaves were brought to the United States and South America (most notably, Brazil, which imported more slaves than any other country), they left their elaborate wood and ivory combs behind. Without combs, shampoos, scissors or they felt they had little choice but to cover their heads in rags or hack off their hair as best as they could, close to the head. The only shears available were those used for sheep and other animals.

Scalp disease and hair damage were prevalent. Sometimes cornmeal was used to clean dirt and oil from the hair, and lard was used in an attempt to protect and soothe the scalp. Sometimes kerosene was rubbed through the hair with rags, or sulfur was used.

One of the earliest methods for straightening hair involved heating a piece of flannel over an open fire, oiling the hair with lard and pulling strands of hair through the hot flannel. Knowledge of braiding techniques survived, and sometimes hair was braided up, under the rags that were used to cover the hair and protect it from the follies of working in cotton fields.

CULTURAL SEGREGATION

Around this time, the Chinese, who often wore their hair in long pigtails, were used as cheap labor to build the railroads. Between 1848, when the U.S. acquired California, and 1869, when the transcontinental railroad was completed, Chinese immigrants, who were not permitted to become citizens, were frequency harassed because of their hair. Westerners, who had heard the Chinese believed that they could not get into "heaven" if their pigtails were cut off (never mind that Shintoists and Buddhists don't believe in "heaven"), would cut off their long braids as cruel sport. In 1882 the Chinese Exclusion Act prevented immigration; later quotas were established, which were not eliminated until 1965. Because of this, Asian beauty care became segregated and was frequently a home-care situation, just as it was for Africans.

After the Civil War ended in 1865, former slaves turned to blacksmith's tools, which were heated at the kitchen stove or fireplace and used as crude straightening irons. Thus the birth of the kitchen or home hairdresser came about. Later blacks began to open their own salons and barber shops. Needless to say, they could not patronize "white" salons and Caucasian hairdressers had neither the desire nor the education to service non-Caucasian clients.

THE DEVELOPMENT OF PRODUCTS FOR CURLY HAIR

Early products used by former-slave barbers were fats, oils and petroleum products. From the turn of the century through the 1950s, the emphasis was on forcing curly hair into a straight configuration. Hair growers and straighteners were introduced in the early 1900s. Many African Americans created their own products, selling concoctions that were developed on kitchen stoves from door to door.

EARLY PIONEERS

Pierre Toussaint, a Haitian-born barber who died in 1853, was recently exhumed from his resting place in a lower Manhattan cemetery, and there is talk about making him a saint. Supposedly, Toussaint's owner freed him (at an unusually early date), but he stayed on to care for his impoverished former owner's widow, supporting her with his hairdressing trade. Barclay Street, where he was buried, was renamed Pierre Toussaint Square; shortly after that, Pierre Toussaint Shampoo turned up at a nearby East Village shop, Little Ricky's.

During Reconstruction, barber shops became the place where men congregated to share news and exchange ideas. For many former slaves, who were just learning to read, barber-shop conversations were the primary source of information. African-American beauty schools sprang up and often doubled as social centers. Some served as hotels, since blacks were not

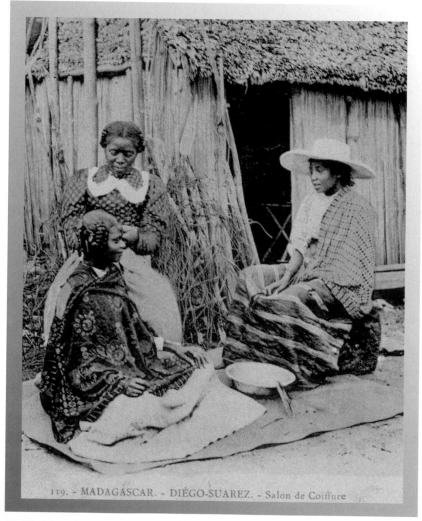

119. - MADAGASCAR. - DIÉGO-SUAREZ. - Salon de Coiffure

FIGURE 2.4
Women dressing their hair. Photographer unknown, ca. 1910; National Museum of African Art, Eliot Elisofon Photographic Archives, Smithsonian Institution.

permitted to stay elsewhere in town.

Throughout this time, many pioneers in beauty culture emerged. Detroit-based historian Vernice Mark provided much of the following information on these early African-American trailblazers.

Annie Turnbo Pope Malone

One school that served as a center of social activity was Poro College, established in St. Louis by Annie Turnbo Pope Malone. Around 1900, Annie, who had never finished high school, began to study chemistry and developed a product called "Wonderful Hair Grower." In 1906 she copyrighted the trade-name "Poro," adapting the slogan, "It Blazes the Trail and Still it Leads."

She traveled throughout the south, promoting her product, settled in St. Louis and began to train young girls in the beauty field. If the girls stayed with her for five years, they received a diamond ring.

By 1918 she moved into the building that became known as Poro College, at the corner of St. Ferdinand and Pendleton Avenues. Poro College grew to hold classrooms, barber shops and a dormitory. At the height of the school's success, Mrs. Malone employed 175 people in the beauty trade, and in 1924 she traveled to Europe to study beauty culture techniques and methods in those countries.

Throughout her life, she gave monetary gifts to a variety of institutions, and in 1945 the St. Louis Orphan's Home Building Fund named its home the Annie Malone Children Home, honoring her for a 10,000 dollar bestowment.

Chuck Berry was one of the many graduates of the St. Louis Poro School of Beauty Culture. He might have been a great cosmetician, but when he was brought to Chess Records in 1955 by Muddy Waters, he turned an old fiddle tune called "Ida Red" into "Maybellene," and a legend was born. While many think Maybellene referred to his beauty-school background, Berry once told a reporter that, as a child, he'd known a cow by that name. (Poro College no longer exists, but its name lives on in the Poro Beauty Salon in St. Louis.)

Madame C. J. Walker

While many African-American barber shops created their own hair oils and products, the most well-known pioneer of hair-care products exclusively for African Americans is Madame C.J. Walker. Born in 1867 in Delta, Louisiana, Sarah Breedlove was orphaned at seven, married at fourteen and widowed at twenty. Sarah McWilliams then married Charles J. Walker, and spend much of her early life as a laundress, earning $1.50 a day. She began developing hair-care products and selling them door-to-door around 1910, and she developed a straightening comb that replaced pull tongs, which she sold along with a hair-growth formula. *Hair growth* is a misleading term; most of these formulations "stretched" the hair, making it appear longer and straighter.

Madame Walker moved her office from city to city and formally established a company in 1911. She continued to expand her line, offering "Tetter Salve," a scalp-treatment product, and opening a beauty school. She produced the first line of cosmetics for black women and eventually employed hundreds of salespeople. The newsletter that she produced for her sales-force included sales tips and a column entitled "Concentrated Wisdom," which provided personal inspirations such as, "Aim for your goal," and "To improve yourself, improve by example." She even authored an instructional book, in which a chapter on bobbed hair recommends that you cut the style to suit the patron's features. It may be the first reference to individualizing a hair-cut.

Throughout the years, she continued to develop her product line and her system of beauty culture education. The "Walker System" eventually came to be taught in Madame C.J. Walker Colleges, located in several cities.

Always keeping control of her company and her money, Madame Walker eventually built a half-million-dollar mansion in Irvington-on-the-Hudson, New York. Her friend the great singer Enrico Caruso named it "Villa Lewaro," for her daughter, Lelia Walker Robinson. It was supposedly furnished for an amount in excess of 350,000 dollars—a virtual fortune at the time.

When Madame C.J. Walker died in 1919, she was eulogized as the richest woman of her race, and many called her the first black millionaire. Her daughter sold Villa Lewaro in 1930, but the company Madame Walker established continued throughout the 1960s, offering over seventy-five different products at its pinnacle.

Sarah Spencer Washington

Sarah Spencer Washington was born some twenty-six years after the Emancipation Proclamation, and around 1914 began her career in beauty culture. She graduated from Norfolk Mission College, studied beauty culture in York, Pennsylvania, and went on to study chemistry at Columbia University. Better prepared educationally than Madame Walker or Annie Malone, she made her mark helping scores of African-American women find financial independence as beauticians.

In 1918 she established her business in Atlantic City, New Jersey, teaching beauty culture during the day and selling her own products at night. Her company, Apex News and Hair Company, used groups of agents, who demonstrated and sold her products. It became the foundation for Apex schools. These schools, which eventually dotted the nation coast-to-coast, graduated thousands of new cosmeticians. Even today, many tell the story of how Madame Washington, as she came to be known, refused to purchase machinery to increase production during the depression, opting instead to retain hundreds of workers who performed tasks manually.

The National Beauty Culture League

One of the oldest and most prestigious beauty organizations in the world is the National Beauty Culturists League (NBLC). Organized on October 1, 1919, in Philadelphia, by R.V. Randolph, S.L. Latimer, E.R. Cargel, M. Paris and B. Tolliver, it was incorporated in 1920 under the laws of the State of Delaware. It was established to further beauty education, advance high standards of conduct, seek beneficial legislation and unify African-American hairdressers.

In 1944, at the NBLC convention in Philadelphia, the National Institute of Cosmetology was established to provide intensive education prior to the convention. Cordelia Greene Johnson founded the institute. Twenty-four students attended the first session in 1944; in 1976 in the Bahamas, 802 students attended.

Throughout the years, the NBLC fought to eliminate segregation on boards of beauty control, provided scholarships to hundreds of aspirants and continued to advance the causes of African-American hairdressers. Today the Institute and the NBLC, headquartered in Washington, D.C., offer annual five-day intensive workshops, a university extension program and a doctoral program with college credits. It is the only known organization offering a Doctorate in the profession; it is also the oldest beauticians' and cosmetologists' organization in the United States.

HAIR STRAIGHTENING

During the 1920s, 1930s and 1940s, pressing the hair with a "straightening comb" or pull tongs became a bi-weekly ritual in African-American homes. Press and curl techniques permitted a variety of styles, including marcel or fingerwaves, upsweeps, French rolls, chignons, Dutch bobs, pompadours and ponytails. Caucasians, who once sat in a tortuous perm machine enduring the smoking and burning of the equipment, switched to the cold wave, which was introduced by the Zotos Corporation in the 1930s.

The 1940s marked the advent of early chemical hair straighteners. During this time, the primary method for straightening hair was to use lye, and it was men, not women, who used the products. The lye was mixed with water and an egg to dissolve the lye crystals and create a thick mixture that could be applied to the hair. Often white potato flour was added in an attempt to cut the burning, but scalp burns and hair l,oss were still a frequent result. The movie *Malcolm X* portrays this painful process realistically, emphasizing the agonizing wait to remove the product. Early straightened styles were called "konked" hair, and one early straightening product was called "Konkaleen."

Through the early 1940s, hair preparations continued to be kitchen brews that had varying measures of efficacy. When finger-waves came into style the stylist or barber had to mold in "memory waves" while the lye product did its work. This definitely demanded gloves, yet some did not use them, in deference to the client, who suffered through the process. Roger Simon, who perfected the early konk fingerwave process, went on to marry Ethel Waters and open a barber shop with comedian Redd Foxx in the 1970s.

TODAY'S PIONEERS

In 1946 Nathaniel Bronner, Sr., formed Bronner Brothers in Atlanta, Georgia. His sister had opened a beauty shop in 1937, and Bronner started selling Apex hair oil, which he took along on his paper route. Today the company has diversified, with beauty supply stores, innumerable products, the Cottonwood Spa and Motel in Cottonwood, Alabama, and *Upscale* magazine, which enjoys national distribution.

In the 1950s commercial hair straighteners were introduced to permanently straighten curly hair. These greatly improved relaxers made it possible for an even greater variety of styles.

Hispanic and Latino men sometimes used similar preparations as those used by African Americans to create the slicked back looks seen at the height of Mambo days. Later, Brylcreem, Vitalis and Wildroot were used to weigh the hair down and keep it back when possible. These three products, more than any other, gave birth to the term "greasers," which was used to label boys with slicked back hair and wild lifestyles, who imitated Elvis Presley.

HISPANIC HOME STYLES

Like African Americans, Hispanics found that there were no products in the mainstream market that met their needs. They developed a variety of creative home-brewed treatments—many of which are now making a resurgence with the return to "natural" and herbal-based products. While during the 1940s and 1950s there were barber shops for men, women turned to home hairdressers, who spoke Spanish and understood their beauty demands. Cubans, Dominicans and Puerto Ricans, who entered the U.S. in large numbers at somewhat different times, worked within their own communities. Cubans, who left their country during Castro's rise to power and frequently settled in Miami, often hid their jewels in their hair to get them out of the country.

The products used and home remedies created were sometimes based on country of origin. However, many different groups of Hispanics arrived at the same solutions. Balmer Galindez, who conducted original research for this book, interviewed many Spanish-speaking stylists who reported that through the 1960s, Hispanics used techniques that were developed decades earlier. Their ingenuity, creativity and determination to have their beauty needs met is evident in the innovative techniques that he discovered.

Relaxers were made using lye, potassium and soap shavings. First the lye was boiled and set to cool. Then soap shavings were added, along with extracted potato juice, which was intended to make the formula gentler and prevent scalp burns. Petroleum was used to base the scalp before the mixture was applied. Other relaxer additives, such as cinnamon sticks, were intended to strengthen the hair. Another hair strengthener was created by boiling the sole of a shoe. The water was used in a relaxer formula or was used alone as a hair treatment.

To create a vibrant haircolor, the bark of the mahogany tree was boiled and mixed with chamomile, cinnamon and an herb called "campeche." For the client who wanted her hair bleached, bleach was made with straight potassium, soap shavings and peroxide. The mixture was extremely strong and required a two-day wait before toning, lest scalp burns result.

Hair was often hot combed; when it was roller set for control, it required the use of a setting lotion. Just a few included a gelatin and water mixture, a mixture of sugar and water or the application of beer that had been allowed to go flat overnight. The hair was set in small sections and wrapped around long, torn strips of paper bag. This technique created ringlets made popular by child star Shirley Temple and was popular with children.

To straighten hair or make a set last longer, the setting lotion was applied and hair was wrapped around an emptied, washed can that once held tomato juice. Both ends of the can were removed, and it was held in place with bobby pins. The hair was covered under a silk scarf until the cans could be removed. Pin curls and fingerwaves were also popular options.

With harsh lyes being used, hair condition was an important beauty issue. Home conditioners used by Hispanic hairdressers are still recommended by consumer beauty magazines in all markets today. These include olive oil mixed with herbs; coconut oil, which was created by frying the meat of the coconut until only oil remained; mashed and strained avocados; and whipped eggs.

Relaxers Improve

Among the first companies to perfect the relaxer were Summit Laboratories, founded in 1959 by three entrepreneurs, and Johnson products, founded by George E. Johnson in 1954. Johnson had previously worked for the Fuller Products Company, another entrepreneurial, African-American-owned company. Throughout the 1980s, the company flourished, but in the early 1990s, Johnson and his wife, who had helped build the company from inception, divorced, and the company changed forever. Johnson Products was the first black-owned company to trade on the stock exchange.

PRODUCTS AND PRIDE LEAD TO NEW— AND REDISCOVERED—STYLES

During the 1960s, which were the Motown years, singers like the Supremes influenced hairstyles with their bouffants, flips, teased tops and pageboys. Wigs and falls became popular, and many African-American women used them to achieve longer hair.

While relaxed hair dominated the market for a time, the Afro usurped it during its popularity, which rose in the mid to late 1960s. In the late 1970s, extension braids became an alternative to the Afro. Cornrows, naturals, African locks, relaxed styles and press and curls were all achievable style alternatives. Then the curly perm was born.

The perfected cold wave process allowed curly hair to be retex-turized or rearranged to simulate soft curls. When the Jheri curl appeared, the product name came to stand for the style.

While new product formulations and chemicals allowed curly-haired clients to experience a range of looks, it wasn't until the late 1980s that men and women of all backgrounds began wearing a vast range of styles. Caucasians abandoned the nightly torture of setting hair on the pink plastic or brush rollers that dominated the 1950s and 1960s; the long, straight styles and perms of the 1970s became more diverse. For African Americans, wearing a relaxed style was no longer considered trying to "look white," any more than a Caucasian wearing a perm was trying to "look black." "Cookie-cutter" or stamped-out, identical looks were disappearing.

Natural Hairstyles

Wearing hair that took advantage of its natural texture also became popular. Native Americans began wearing traditional ornamentation—without expulsion from schools; Puerto Rican and other Hispanic women began to enjoy their naturally curly locks without subduing them via roller sets. In the late 1970s, braided styles reappeared and have grown in popularity ever since. Most are based on the ancient art of cornrowing, which is called *canerowing* by West Indians. In modern styles, the hair is either braided without hair additions, or human or synthetic hair is woven into the cornrows, or attached and braided on its own.

The art of cultivating natural locks also reappeared. For years, many associated locks with the "dreadlocks" worn by Rastafarians and West Indians, which are created by allowing the elements to have an effect on hair. But in the 1980s, ancient African techniques for creating cultivated locks re-emerged, giving birth to a whole new professional title: locktician. Lockticians do not use hair additions, but guide curly hair through natural stages of growth until it permanently locks in place. In the modern spelling *locks* often becomes *locs*.

Modern Developments

In 1981 the American Health and Beauty Aids Institute (AHBAI) was founded as a national association of black-owned companies that produce hair -care and cosmetic products for the black consumer. In response to African-American-owned companies losing 30 percent of market share in the 1980s to mass-market companies, the organization introduced the Proud Lady logo, which stands for membership in the organization and the goal of keeping black dollars in the black community.

Braiders and natural hairstylists, who had continued to pass down and perfect techniques from generation to generation, grew in numbers and popularity throughout the 1970s; in the 1980s they began to demand the right to separate licensing. They became part of a cultural revival that rediscovered history, and today they are redefining African-American beauty.

Since natural hairstylists do not use chemicals and have a completely different philosophy about hair, many do not want to be constrained by cosmetology regulations, which were written in the 1930s. Licensing regulations that required graduation from a cosmetology school were intended to protect clients from improper chemical usage, and make no sense to the natural or "cultural hairstylist." In addition, cosmetology schools do not teach the braiding techniques that natural stylists needed to know.

A Distinct and Separate Profession

By the 1990s, states began to create separate specialty licenses for braiders, lockticians and natural hairstylists, who deliver very different services from cosmetologists. Braiders in Washington, D.C., fought for separate licensing and won it after a ten-year political battle; licensing for natural hairstyling has also passed in New York. While some believed that natural or cultural hairstylists should not be subjected to any licensing procedure, for others the license represents recognition of the profession and an upgrading of standards. It also permits the development of a separate curriculum that, at last, will teach what natural stylists need to know.

Today, braid artists, lockticians and cultural hairstylists work out of their homes and in numerous salons across the U.S., where the elaborate styles they create are astonishingly intricate works of beauty, much like the braids and locks of early African tribes. In fact, most of the techniques they use are based on almost-lost, rediscovered arts.

In 1994 the International Braiders Network, based in Brooklyn, New York, held the first ever natural hair-care conference. The show highlighted historical and cultural traditions of black hair care.

CONCLUSION

It is apparent from history that hairstyling always was and still is a very social and political issue. In America, the unrealized ideal of personal freedom and choice has resulted in a sometimes superficial approach to hair. However, as America develops into a new multicultural society, the time is ripe for a "hair revolution" that embraces and touts all the rich history and diversity of hairstyling, and the multitudinous statements it can make.

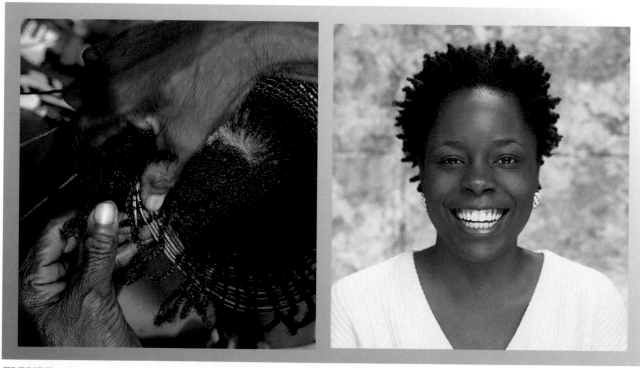

FIGURE 2.5
Mangbetu chief's principal wife having hair styled in traditional manner, Madje village, Zaire. Photo: Eliot Elisofon, 1970; National Museum of African Art, Eliot Elisofon Photographic Archives, Smithsonian Institution.

FIGURE 2.6
Modern style.

LOCKS 'ROUND THE CLOCK

3000 B.C.	Egyptians wore braided styles, wigs with shaved heads, used henna
2500 B.C.	Hair ornamentation popular in many parts of the world
2000 B.C.	Braids worn by nomadic groups in China
1400 B.C.	Ungents and waxes used to dress hair
500 B.C.	Heated tools used for hairstyling
400 B.C..	Beard shaving popular
55 B.C.	Men's hair primarily long in many parts of the world
27 B.C.	The Gauls dye their hair red
300 A.D.	Beards back in vogue
1090	European men wear long locks, beards, moustaches
1520	King Henry VIII introduces short hair to England
1630	European men and women wear long locks; women's styles are wider
1680	European men dye their hair, wear powdered wigs, false beards
1820	Dressed hair popular in the U.S. Center parts, chignons, knots
1930s	Permanent waving widespread
1940s	Fingerwaves and konked styles
1950s	Relaxed styles, short cuts, bleaching, slicked looks for men
1960s	Long, straight hair; the Afro, wigs and falls, the Bob
1970s	The shag, perms and Jheri curls, braids and extensions
1980s	Spikes, waves, crimps, weaves, braids, punk styles
1984	Mousse introduced by L'Oreal as "Free Hold"
1995	The freeze, fades, casual styles in all lengths, bald heads

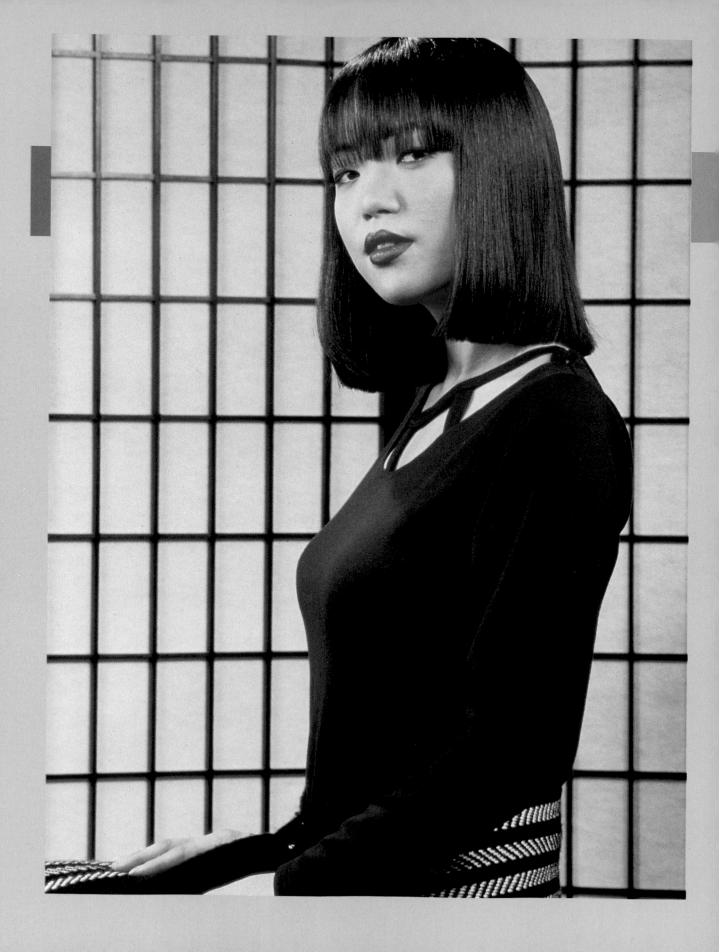

Hair Structure and Its Varieties

The modern hairstylist looks at hair as a fiber that is the medium for his or her art. The primary variances are in hair shape, diameter and color. Shape determines curl configuration, and shape is dependent on genetic coding, according to geneticists. Just as the gene for dark-colored hair is dominant, while the gene for blonde hair is recessive, the gene for crimped or extremely curly hair is dominant over the gene for curly, wavy or straight hair.

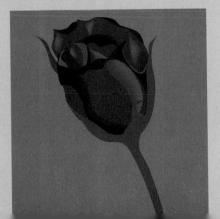

The precise mechanism that creates curl is not thoroughly understood, although many scientists think it has to do with the shape of the hair bulb, which is produced by the matrix cells. (Previously, the follicle was suspected, but the soft keratin of the follicle takes the shape of the hair within it.)

According to one theory, golf-shaped bulbs periodically displace the center of cell division, resulting in a different keratin formation. Because of uneven cellular division, the bond responsible for curl forms at an angle. The sharper the angle, the stronger the observed curl pattern.

If you understand hair's structure and its reactions to cosmetic or chemical services, you will be able to successfully predict the outcome of each service. Therefore a review is in order.

HAIR COMPOSITION

Hair is composed primarily of the protein keratin. Its chemical composition includes carbon, oxygen, hydrogen, nitrogen and sulfur. While there is disagreement about the precise proportions present, it is believed that darker hair contains more carbon and less oxygen than lighter-colored hair; light-colored hair contains more oxygen and sulfur.

Haircolor originates in melanosomes, which contain varying degrees of pigment and have four stages of development. According to a 1980 report by Redken Laboratories, African hair contains more stage 4 melanosomes, which have the most dense pigment, while Caucasians—particularly blondes—have more stage 1 and 2 melanosomes in their hair than stage 4 melanosomes. Stage 2 melanosomes contain less melanin; during this stage, there is often no evidence of melanin in the melanosomes at all. Also naturally curly hair contains more hydrogen.

HAIR STRUCTURE

Hair has a root and a shaft. The root is enclosed within the follicle and the shaft is visible to the eye. Most commonly, one follicle houses a single hair; however a single follicle can hold as many as three hairs, which affects density. (Fig. 3.1)

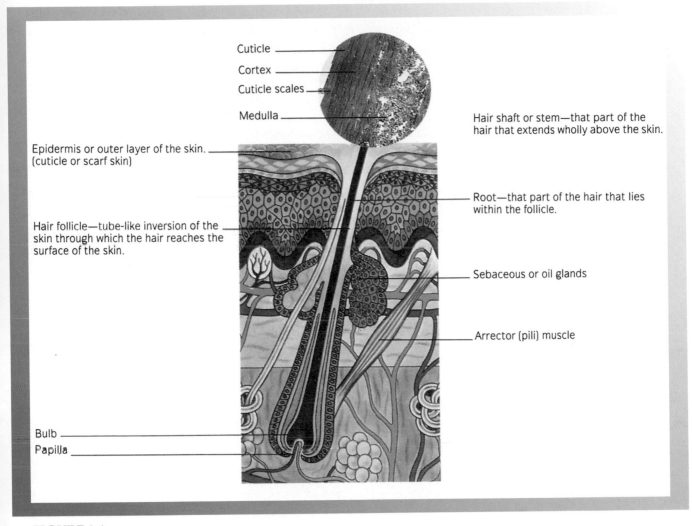

Cuticle

Cortex

Cuticle scales

Medulla

Hair shaft or stem—that part of the hair that extends wholly above the skin.

Epidermis or outer layer of the skin. (cuticle or scarf skin)

Root—that part of the hair that lies within the follicle.

Hair follicle—tube-like inversion of the skin through which the hair reaches the surface of the skin.

Sebaceous or oil glands

Arrector (pili) muscle

Bulb

Papilla

FIGURE 3.1
Cross section of hair and skin.

INTERNAL STRUCTURE

The follicle, the bulb and the papilla are the primary root structures. The **follicle** is a pocket-like structure that encases the root. Just below the follicle are sebaceous or oil glands. These produce sebum, which gives hair its luster and keeps the scalp supple. Sebum is nature's "natural moisturizer."

The hair **bulb** is a club-shaped structure that holds the lower portion of the root. The lower part of the bulb is hollowed out to fit over the papilla.

The **papilla** is a cone-shaped elevation at the very bottom of the follicle that fits into the bulb. Here blood is supplied and hair growth occurs. Through the papilla nourishment reaches the bulb.

Given this progression, you can see how anything that enters the bloodstream can potentially affect hair and its growth. Drugs, vitamins and other chemicals can leave traces within the cortex, where they will affect chemical services. For instance, calcium supplements, commonly used among women, can create problems when chemically reconstructing hair. Additionally, over- or underproduction of sebum can result in oily hair, dandruff or oily dandruff.

EXTERNAL STRUCTURE

The visible hair shaft is composed of three layers: an outer cuticle layer, a middle cortex layer and an inner medulla. The number of cuticle layers and their degree of compactness vary among groups of people and individuals, as does the size or diameter of the cortex. The medulla may be absent in very fine hair.

The Cuticle

The **cuticle** is comprised of overlapping layers of flat cells. These translucent, scale-like cells point away from the scalp, toward the ends. The cuticle's biological purpose is protective, and the arrangement and shape of the scales vary among individuals and hair types.

The cuticle is responsible for the hair's resistance to or absorption of liquids, or its porosity. It is believed that extremely curly, African hair has more cuticle layers than straight, European hair, and Asian hair is also made up of more cuticle layers than straight, European hair. However, the world's foremost forensic scientists have noted that markers, such as the structure of the bones, teeth and hair, which were once used by them to identify bodies by race, are less and less useful. According to them, the notion of racial "purity," particularly in the United States, is obsolete, and mixing among the races has made it nearly impossible for them to determine race from a skeleton that has hair left on it.

For the hairdresser, the precise number of cuticle layers in hair is not as significant as how compact they are. (Even twelve layers are thinner than the eye can see.) The more compact the cuticle, the less porous hair will be and the more difficult it will be for the chemicals used in perming and relaxing to penetrate the cuticle. This is known as *resistance*.

Extremely curly hair, thought to have more cuticle layers, will relax relatively quickly, because it is more porous. Some believe that the hair thins out as it bends and that high porosity exists at each bend. Wavy hair is considered harder to relax than super-curly hair because the cuticle is more compact. Very fine, straight hair and coarse, thick hair can also have compact cuticles.

Since chemical services, mechanical mistreatment and thermal damage can all affect porosity, it is best to test any hair to determine the porosity level before you make assumptions about hair types. Once you know how resistant the hair will be to the penetration of liquids, you can adjust the strength of your product or the timing accordingly. Of course, the use of stronger chemicals and longer processing times means that post-service conditioning is essential. Keep in mind that the hair analysis and the consultation are the most important procedures for achieving the desired results. During these procedures you will make decisions about product selection and timing of the service.

The Cortex

The second layer of hair and the one that concerns cosmetologists the most is the **cortex.** The cortex is comprised of interwoven fibers that are arranged in a helix configuration. The cortex gives hair its strength, moisture, elasticity, resiliency and curl.

Most melanocytes are contained in the cortex; therefore, this is where color originates. In general, a smaller-diameter cortex means that products will act faster once they've penetrated the cuticle. A smaller cortex also makes hair more susceptible to heat damage. Sulfur and hydrogen bonds, which are affected by chemicals, are located in the cortex.

A cross section of the cortex shows that, in general, straight hair is usually round, wavy hair is oval and extremely curly hair is flat. While the shape of the hair shaft—round, oval or flat—was once considered a distinguishing characteristic of race, hair from curly to straight and textures from fine to dense exist in different races and nationalities, as well as in those who are of mixed heritage.

The Medulla

In the innermost portion of the hair shaft lies the **medulla.** The medulla is a loose arrangement of cells that comprise the smallest portion of the hair shaft. In animals the medulla serves as part of an insulating mechanism; in humans its role is not understood. Some claim it serves no purpose; others believe it is a genetic remnant of evolution; still others think it excretes materials from the hair and serves as a source of moisture and nutrients.

The medulla can be destroyed by chemical services and physical damage. Sometimes it is present only in hair below the surface level. It is believed that the medulla may be absent in very fine hair and the downy hairs that grow on the body.

COMPOSITION, STRUCTURE AND MODERN SCIENCE

As often happens, the more you learn the more you have to relearn. The growth mechanism of hair seemed rather straightforward until an article appeared in the *New York Times* a few years ago, reporting the discovery that the source of new hair cells is not at the base of the hair, as long thought, but farther up the follicle, just below the scalp. Does this mean the cells move downward and take root? Who knows. While this may not concern you as a cosmetologist (yet), it greatly interests those who are seeking a cure for baldness.

Scientists at the University of Miami have also discovered two types of protein, one present in the glands of bald men and the other in the glands of men who have hair. Having isolated the factor that controls production of these proteins and converted one protein to the other in test tubes, the scientific team is face with the quandary of how to use this converter in humans. But don't get too excited; it's one thing to make genetic changes in a test tube and quite another to make use of the knowledge in humans.

However, two relatively new scientific revelations about hair structure and composition are useful to the cosmetologist right now. One involves how hair holds a history of all drug use and diet; the other involves the effect of hard mineral water on the hair.

HAIR STRUCTURE AND MEDICATIONS

For years, manufacturers and cosmetologists debated what went wrong when suddenly a perm or relaxer didn't take or haircolor didn't come out right. Chemists frequently attributed these results to stylist error, but reports persisted from stylists who had been performing the same service on the same client for years and suddenly experienced a different result.

Labs used by the F.B.I. were among the first to discover that the cortex holds traces of drugs. (Cocaine in particular can be found in the cortex and in the cuticle, where it is easily separated by placing hair in a warm alcohol bath.) With this discovery came the realization that prescription medications and vitamins deposit in the cortex, as does a history of diet. Biophysicist Taft Toribara determined levels of zinc and mercury from the hair of 400-year-old bodies found frozen in Alaska, indicating which times of year they ate red meat and which times of year they ate fish. He also discovered a low zinc content in the hair of an alcoholic.

Since hair grows at a rate of half-an-inch (or one centimeter) a month, an inch will reveal about two-and-a half months of history. Very little is known about how various medications housed in the cortex affect hair services (or deplete essential vitamins enough to affect hair), but many stylists claim that if clients take iron supplements, the supplements can affect haircolor. Given the discovery that the hair holds many secrets, if the result of your services suddenly changes, you might consider asking clients about the medications they're taking, changes in diet or vitamin supplements.

Effects of Medication and Chemicals on Hair

To make the best use of this information, recognize that chemicals can leave traces in the cortex, where they could possibly affect services such as perming and relaxing. As a matter of course, have new clients fill out a card that includes the prescription drugs they are taking, as well as supplements such as calcium and iron. Then keep track of the success of your chemical services. If results suddenly change, refer to your client card and ask the client if any of the data has changed. Over time, you may identify information that can be used with all clients.

Drugs used in chemotherapy treatment are among the most likely to affect hair services. They frequently result in hair loss, but there are occasions when a client who has not yet experienced dramatic hair loss may not reveal that he or she is undergoing chemotherapy. If your service suddenly fails, you must use sound judgment about what you ask your client and how. If a client indicates that his or her use of prescription drugs has not changed, respect the right to privacy. Re-check all your steps, and if you cannot determine the cause of the failure, refrain from attempting a repeat for at least six weeks.

While at one time physicians recommended using a tourniquet applied to the scalp or an ice bath to prevent chemotherapy drugs from reaching hair follicles, these methods not only cause discomfort but do not prevent hair loss. Do not recommend or attempt them.

Sometimes you can feel or see the presence of medications. If the hair shaft feels coated or brittle, or if hair that has always been gray has a color cast that did not come from haircolor, medication may be the cause.

HAIR COMPOSITION AND HARD WATER

There are two theories about hair and its electrical charge. The first is that hair has a negative electrical charge. While no one who claims this knows why, one theory is that since most toxins have a positive charge, the body developed a negative charge as a defense system to repel them. When you comb your hair and a negative electron jumps onto the comb, static electricity results.

The second theory holds that the hair shaft has particular sites of both positive and negative charges and that damaged hair has more negatively charged sites.

Regardless of which theory is correct, positively charged minerals are attracted to the negatively charged hair (or sites) like magnets. As a result, when a client shampoos her hair in hard, mineral-laden water, over time she will experience a mineral buildup. Depending on where your client lives, the minerals that build up could be copper, iron, calcium or other trace elements. (Soft water does not result in a mineral buildup.)

Treating Buildup

Mineral buildup can affect all chemical services; therefore, it is advisable to remove it before a chemical service. There are many products on the market for this purpose. If water is just slightly hard, a vinegar rinse may be effective. Remove the minerals and your chemical services will take better and the color truer.

If you client has been shampooing in mineral water over a period of time and you have never removed the buildup before, treat the service as though it were a first-time service. Don't rely on what always worked. The timing of a perm or a relaxer will be most likely be shorter; haircolor will be brighter. Red shades in particular will be far more vibrant because larger red molecules will have had less penetration in the past, when mineral buildup hindered them.

Salon owners who live in hard-water areas would be well advised to invest in water softeners to combat mineral buildup and to encourage clients to do the same for their homes. However, since many cities use more than one water supply, it wouldn't be unusual for a salon to have moderately soft water and its clients to have hard water at home. Test the water with a test strip and have your client do the same before making an investment in a water softener. You may find that you'll use fewer cleansing products in the long run.

HAIR VARIETIES

It has been said that over fifty variations of hair types have been identified. Curl configurations vary widely, as does hair texture. Texture is usually determined by the diameter of hair, which can be larger or smaller based on the absence or presence of a medulla, a larger or smaller cortex and a greater or fewer number of cuticle layers. Coarse, thick hairs have a larger diameter; fine, thin hairs have a smaller diameter. As we grow older, the cuticle can shrink, making hair finer than it once was.

Given the wide range of hair types within all groups of people, the simplest way to ensure the success of a service is to perform an analysis to determine the hair's curl pattern, texture and density, porosity, tensile strength, pH and natural growth patterns and directions. All this information will be used to determine the strength of relaxer to use, the timing of a perm or the likelihood that hair cannot withstand a particular chemical service. With speed and practice, you should be able to determine these factors in a matter of minutes, during the consultation.

CURL CONFIGURATION

Take an individual hair and observe the curl pattern. Is is extremely curly, moderately curly, slightly wavy or straight? Super-curly hair looks like a coil, medium curl has an *S*-shaped pattern, slightly wavy hair has an elongated curl and straight hair is not always as obvious as you might think. While some hair is super straight, other "straight" hair has a slight bend.

If you're uncertain, spritz hair lightly with water, pull it straight, using only as much tension as required, and observe it as it dries and reverts to its natural curl configuration. Also examine the hair to determine whether the curl configuration exists uniformly or changes. Often medium-curly hair can be very curly at the nape and at the hairline.

This information will be extremely important when choosing a relaxer strength and determining timing. Super-curly hair will relax best with a regular or medium strength relaxer; elongated curl patterns require a super-strength relaxer to penetrate the hair's more compact cuticle. When perming Asian hair, the biggest mistake made is over-processing to compensate for the compact cuticle. In general, it's best to use a stronger perm that works faster, putting less chemical stress on the hair in the long run.

TEXTURE AND DENSITY

Examine the hair to determine if it is coarse, medium or fine. Look for variations in texture around the head and at the hairline, which is often finer. In general, the coarser the hair's texture, the greater its internal strength and resistance to change. Extremely coarse textures can also be more porous, if the hair is curly or damaged. In general,

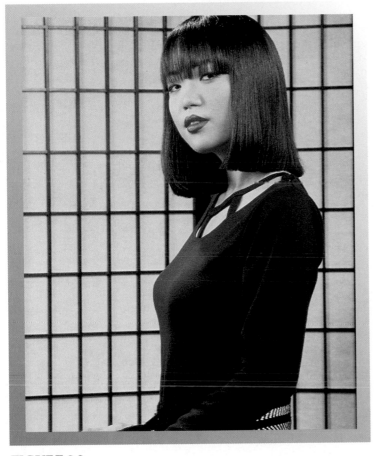

FIGURE 3.2
Observe hair texture and density. Hair: Denice Hansen; Photo: J.D. Chielli for John Paul Mitchell Systems.

coarse hair is larger in diameter; fine hair is small in diameter.

Fine or small-diameter hair will process more quickly than coarse or large diameter hair, unless porosity becomes a variable. Then porosity matters more. Porous, coarse hair will process faster than fine, non-porous hair. Remember, "P" (for porous) comes before "T" (texture) when determining processing times.

Next note the abundance of hair. How many strands exist per square inch? This determines density. A client can have fine hair but lots of it or coarse hair that is sparsely distributed. The hair's density will affect the final results of a perm or any other service. For example, regardless of its texture, if hair distribution is extremely sparse, a perm could result in too much of the scalp showing. If it is thin but not excessively so, do not use large sections during perming or you won't get proper curl formation near the scalp. However, if hair is fine but there's lots of it, you'll want to take smaller sections when cutting. If hair is both coarse and dense, use the smallest sections of all.

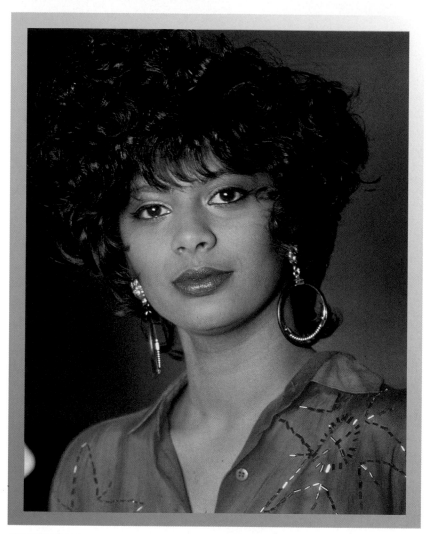

FIGURE 3.3
Examine hair texture and density before perming in order to guarantee proper curl formation. Hair: Fran Cotter for John Paul Mitchell Systems; Photo: Jack Cutler.

POROSITY

Hair that is very porous grabs color quickly and absorbs chemicals rapidly. If hair is too porous, it may need a filler before coloring or regular conditioning treatments—and a vacation from exposure to heat—before a chemical service. Additionally, porous hair will "frizz up" more easily in humid weather. Hair damage is directly related to porosity; the more porous the hair, the greater the damage possibilities.

To test for porosity, comb a small section of hair and hold the ends firmly with the thumb and index finger of one hand while you slide the fingers of the opposite hand from ends to the roots. If your fingers do not slide easily or if the cuticle ruffles up, the hair is porous. The more the hair ruffles, the more porous it is. Overly porous hair is often identifiable by sight. It is frayed, dry, fragile and brittle.

Other tests for porosity include:

◆ Cut the dry hair. If the scissors meet little resistance, hair is porous.
◆ Squeeze the hair with your fingers and release it. If it is porous, it will have little or no spring to it.
◆ Spritz the hair with water. If it absorbs the water quickly and wets easily, the hair is porous.

Hair that has a very compact cuticle will be resistant to chemical absorption. It will not be porous at all. Resistant hair may include coarse, straight hair; gray hair; coarse, wavy hair; or any texture that cannot be easily straightened with medium-strength relaxer. Resistant hair may require stronger products or longer processing times for curls, perms and haircolor.

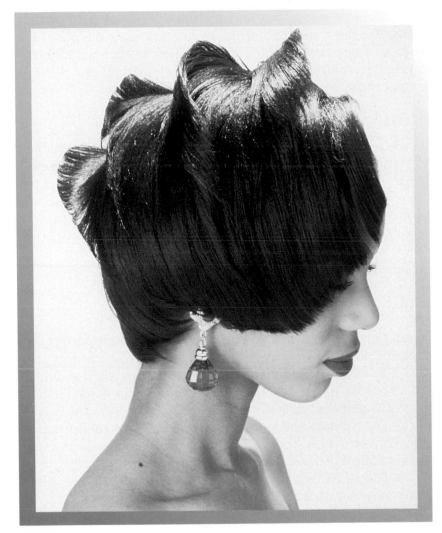

FIGURE 3.4
Creating unique styles requires pre-analysis of growth patterns and hair condition. Hair: Laurence E. Nunes for John Paul Mitchell Systems; Photo: Paul Edwards.

TENSILE STRENGTH

Tensile strength indicates the hair's elasticity. To test it, pull a single hair to see how much it stretches before it breaks. Dry hair that is healthy should stretch about one-fifth; or 20 percent, of its length before it breaks. Wet hair stretches 40 to 50 percent of its length before it breaks, if it has good elasticity. Relaxing and perming services can affect tensile strength, because each time the hair's internal bonds are broken and rearranged, some of the bonds remain broken. Rebonding is never a 100 percent proposition.

NATURAL GROWTH PATTERNS AND DIRECTIONS

Move the hair from side to side and observe the growth patterns and directions. Are there cowlicks at the front hairline or whorls at the crown, just above the occipital? The nape often has its own highlyunique growth patterns. You'll want to work with these patterns when you cut the hair and style it.

HAIR pH

Ideally hair should have a pH of 4.8. (About 4.0 to 5.5 is acceptable.) To test hair's pH level, pour a spoonful or two of distilled water over the hair, wait five minutes and "squeeze" the water out onto a pH test strip. The water takes on the hair's pH. If it is above 5.5, the hair is probably drier or weaker than normal.

. . . .

HAIR STRUCTURE AND SERVICES

Understanding hair structure will help you prescribe the correct services, products, home-care regimen and retail products for your clientele. You will know when to perform a relaxing service, which strength of relaxer to use, the appropriate timing and when the hair will not withstand the service.

If you do not understand porosity, texture and curl configuration in particular, you will not be able to build your business with higher-priced chemical services. To heighten your understanding, gather samples of hair of all types and test them in your own home chemistry lab, observing various products as they work.

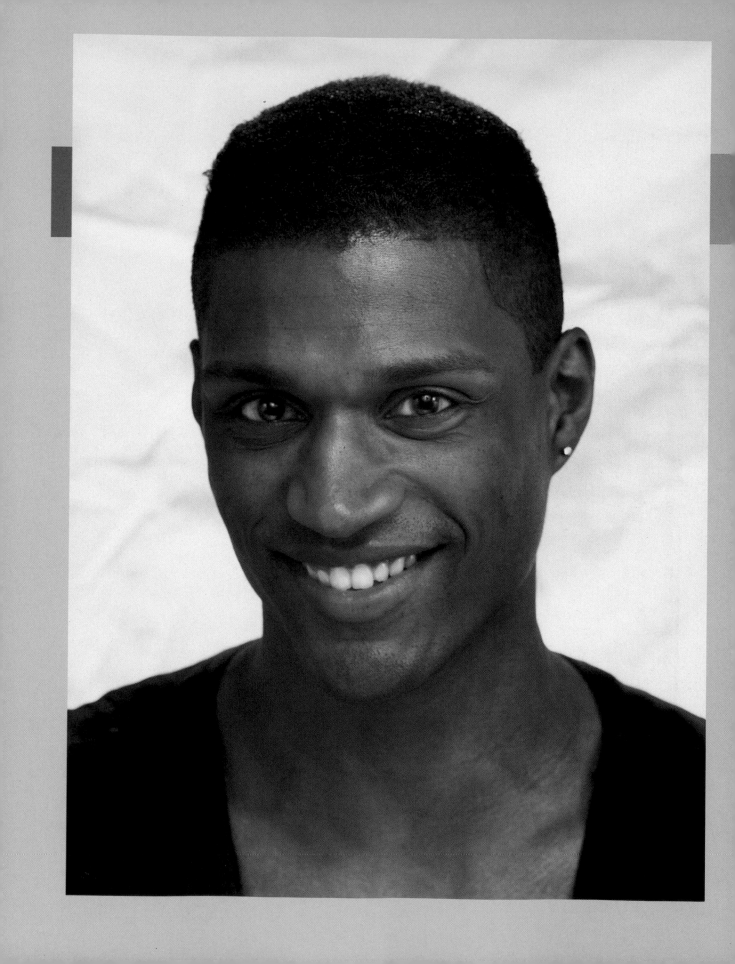

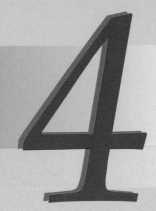

Conducting a Successful Analysis- Based Consultation

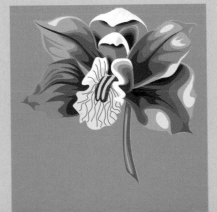

An effective consultation takes a number of factors into account. These are:

◆ The hair analysis. What exists?

◆ A scalp analysis. Does the condition of the scalp preclude any procedures?

◆ Previous services. Which services has the client had in the past and how will they affect a future service?

◆ The client's desires.

◆ What is realistically possible.

◆ Two-way communication. Are you both speaking the same language and understanding one another?

◆ The client's lifestyle. Is the client asking for a style that he or she will never have the time or desire to maintain?

◆ The client's skin tone and eye color. These will help determine the haircolor that will best suit him or her.

◆ The client's personal style. Is she a corporate woman who has a conservative image, or does she favor high-fashion, trendy looks? Does he like a no-fuss look, or is he interested in being able to change his hair to get several different looks?

◆ The ability to arrive at a decision. Can you and the client agree—particularly if his or her desires clash with what's realistically possible?

SALON READINESS

A well-known humorous bumper sticker reads, "I'm a beautician, not a magician." But the accomplished, educated stylist should be able to satisfy every client, even if it means explaining why the hair is too damaged to perform a relaxing service, offering an alternative and making him or her realize you are operating in a professional manner. If you can do this, you can enhance the natural attractiveness of every client, which is an act of artistry, not magic.

When you work in a salon, you face a wide range of challenging situations. Perhaps the most challenging is arriving at a solution that pleases the client. In this respect, your success will depend more on your communication skills than on your technical ability. Clients have great expectations and believe that you can deliver them. But if they cannot realistically have what they want, they won't be disappointed if you can explain why and offer alternatives.

What follows is a detailed look at each step of the analysis-based consultation, which will lead to success with all clients.

THE HAIR ANALYSIS

As soon as you greet your client, begin the hair analysis. Observe all the areas noted in the previous chapter. Check for curl configuration, texture, density, porosity or resistance, tensile strength, natural growth patterns and directions. If you suspect pH will be a factor, test for it at the shampoo bowl. Also look for any signs of breakage. If the ends are split or frayed, a trim or a break from daily thermal styling is in order. However, if breakage occurs mid-strand, there may be chemical damage, in which case you'll want to delay a chemical service and begin a series of reconstructive treatments.

It's always best to see the client's hair before it's shampooed, even with regular clients. (Fig. 4.1) You'll be able to easily re-evaluate porosity each time and observe how well the client is able to maintain his or her hairstyle. It's also easier for the client to indicate to you how long or short the hair should be when it is dry. Additionally, when you see clients before they change into a cape or gown, you'll be able to observe their personal style. Take note of what the client is wearing and his or her preferred approach to fashion.

If this is your client's first visit, make notes on your client record card as you perform the analysis. Other information you'll want to note on the card will emerge as the consultation continues.

THE HAIR TEST

Curly-haired clients use a variety of styling techniques, and you can't always tell by looking if the hair is pressed, relaxed, roller set or chemically

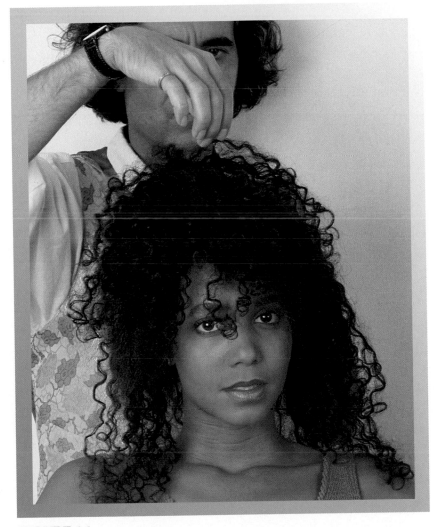

FIGURE 4.1
Before you shampoo or drape the client, analyze her hair and style. Photo: Steven Landis with direction from Vincent and Alfred Nardi of Nardi Salon, New York City, New York.

curled. If you aren't certain if a relaxer or a thio solution is on the hair, use this test:

Mist the hair lightly with water. If it goes straight, it is relaxed. If it curls up, it is chemically curled. If it reverts, it has been pressed.

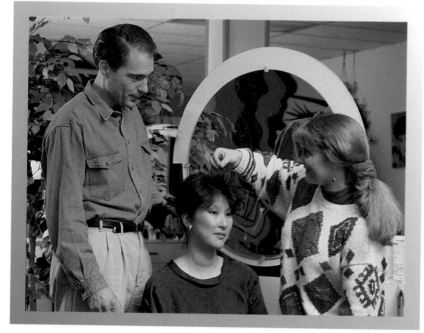

FIGURE 4.2
Performing a professional hair and scalp analysis. Photo: Michael Gallitelli on location at Rielms Hair Salon, Latham, New York.

THE SCALP ANALYSIS

To perform a professional scalp analysis, part the hair into half-inch sections and begin by looking for cuts, abrasions, eruptions or open sores. If any are present, do not proceed with any chemical service. Also check for:

◆ Signs of dry scalp or dandruff.
◆ Signs of excessive oil.
◆ Parasites.
◆ Sparse areas or indication of alopecia.
◆ Flexibility and pliability.

USING THE INFORMATION

If you find any contraindications to the service, refer the client to a dermatologist. The scalp examination is particularly important to the curly-haired client because relaxers are the most caustic chemicals used by cosmetologists. However, no client should be given a perm or haircolor if the scalp is abraded.

◆ If the client has any form of hair additions, look for the tell-tale sign of pin-sized bumps that indicate they are too tight. (Additionally, too-tight braids or hair extensions can result in damage to the hair's root.)
◆ If the scalp is inflexible, do not proceed with a hair addition service. Instead, offer scalp massage and high-frequency treatments. (It is rare that any scalp is too flexible; the more common situation that affects a service decision is a too-tight scalp.)
◆ If the scalp is oily, determine whether it is from overactive sebaceous glands product usage. If the client has applied oil

to the scalp, it is usually dispersed evenly over the head, and some oil will appear on the hair strands.

◆ If the client has a sensitive scalp, you'll want to advise against scratching the scalp with a comb, braiding hair tightly or putting excess mechanical tension on the hair. If the scalp is sensitive but not abraded, select a no-lye relaxer and use a protective base cream; opt for gentler, buffered perms and non-peroxide haircolors when possible. In both cases, keep a close eye on the scalp as the product develops and rinse it off immediately if your client complains of discomfort.

◆ If dry dandruff exists, you can offer scalp treatments. Keep in mind that dandruff is contagious. Sterilize all your tools whenever a client's scalp shows evidence of dandruff, however mild.

PREVIOUS SERVICES

As you examine the hair and scalp, begin to ask the questions about previous services. (Fig. 4.3) Questions of particular importance include:

◆ Which chemical services have you had in the last six months?

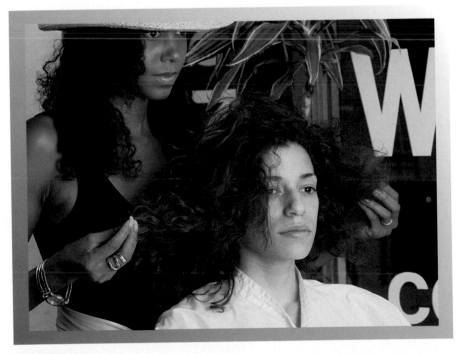

FIGURE 4.3
During her consultation, question the client about previous services. Photo: Steven Landis with direction from Vincent and Alfred Nardi of Nardi Salon, New York City, New York.

◆ How long ago was your last chemical service?
◆ Was a sodium or thio-based relaxer used?
◆ Which type of haircolor product was used?
◆ Have you ever used henna or a metallic dye; if so, when?
◆ When was the last time you had a regrowth touch-up?

Remember, you cannot use a thio-based product if a sodium hydroxide, sodium bromide or calcium hydroxide product remains on the hair. The reverse is also true. If the client has haircolor and now wants a relaxing service, wait until color has been on the hair for a week before relaxing it. Then use a mild-strength relaxer.

Often clients do not consider henna haircolor and won't mention it unless specifically asked, but it can affect your color results. Henna remains in the hair much longer than clients believe and can affect results even after a year. It is very difficult to remove; therefore a strand test is recommended if henna is present. If a colored henna has been used, find out which color and neutralize it during a strand test by using a color opposite on the color wheel. (Red neutralizes green, etc.)

Metallic dyes, which are sold over the counter, must be removed. Their presence is indicated by an unnatural cast to the hair and can sometimes be felt. Hair with a buildup of metallic dye feels rough. Men are more likely to have used metallic dyes than women, because coloring products aimed at men are more likely to contain them.

If a client has received a haircolor service within a week, avoid perms, curls and relaxers, which will lighten the color. Also ascertain if your client has been receiving regular conditioning and scalp treatments before proceeding with any chemical service. If they are warranted, delay the chemical service.

FINE-LINE DECISIONS

If your client wants curl, the hair's natural configuration will determine whether you use a two-step or single-step process. While experience will be your best guide, in general, if the hair has an elongated S-shape, is slightly wavy or straight, you can wrap the hair with water and apply a waving solution. If the client's hair ranges between being extremely curly and having an S-shaped curl, you'll want to straighten the hair first and then rearrange it into the new curl configuration by wrapping with the solution or applying the solution after wrapping or "rodding" the hair.

A question to ask yourself is: Am I creating a curl that's tighter than the client's natural formation, or am I creating a softer, looser one? Often, Middle Eastern, Jewish, Hispanic, African and other clients will present borderline situations. A point to keep in mind is that when possible, avoid additional chemical stress.

This point also applies when hair is straight, coarse and resistant. For less stress, use an alkaline, not an exothermic perm. The reason is that alkaline perms are stronger, but are left on the hair a shorter period of time than exothermic perms, which require heat and additional time.

THE DESIRED LOOK

Most clients will tell you what they want; it is up to you to recommend changes. Listen closely to everything the client says, then repeat the information so you know you are communicating properly. Ask the following questions to determine whether your clients really want what they think they do:

- ◆ How often are you willing to get a (relaxer, color, etc.) touch-up?
- ◆ Will you be coming in for a "root press" (regrowth press) between relaxer touch-ups, or will you do this at home?
- ◆ How often can you come in to have extensions adjusted?
- ◆ Are you considering haircolor?
- ◆ What do want most? (Curl, body, etc.)
- ◆ How will you be styling your hair at home?
- ◆ Which products do you use at home?
- ◆ Do you want the style for a one-time special occasion?
- ◆ What do you like/dislike about your hair?

The answers to all these questions will affect your service decision.

SERVICE LIMITATIONS

Always be honest about how existing factors limit what is realistically possible. A client who has two inches of hair cannot have a French Roll without hair additions. A client with extremely porous or decolorized, damaged hair will not be able to get a relaxing service that day. Permanent haircolor cannot be applied the same day as a relaxer. A highly alkaline shampoo used at home can remove the curl you created, so a service may depend on the client's willingness to change the retail products he or she uses.

If any conditions preclude the requested service and the client insists, suggest a second opinion. Don't damage clients' hair to please them in the short run.

Often clients who have relaxed hair want to change to a chemical curl or vice versa. Explain that regrowth is essential for curl restructuring and that you cannot apply incompatible products over one another without the risk of hair loss. There are other styling options, such as thermal curling, roller setting and pressing, that will give clients the look they want until the hair grows out enough for you to treat the new growth and either cut off the remainder or continue to style it.

The hair's condition and porosity will be the most limiting factors when it comes to making a service decision. Another consideration is the client's age. With age the cuticle shrinks and the hair becomes more fragile. Often skin tone can get lighter or ashy, which will influence your choice of a haircolor. Since 80 percent of people over fifty have some form of arthritis, the client's ability to style his or her own hair also becomes a factor in making a style decision.

If the client is a child, keep in mind that a lifetime of relaxing or curling is not always the best option. Cultural hairstylists often point out that children who have extremely curly hair are the only ones who potentially experience a lifetime of chemical usage. Hairstyles that use the natural texture are ideal for children, although it's the parent with whom you'll be discussing this.

If you're unfamiliar with all the factors that may limit a service decision, return to a basic cosmetology textbook and brush up on the fundamentals.

TWO-WAY COMMUNICATION

To ensure that you and the client are speaking the same language, rely on the universal language of photos. Other tips include:

◆ Repeat back to the client what you heard him or her tell you, to make certain that you truly heard what the client said.

◆ Keep in mind that many African-American clients will say they want a "perm" when what they want is a relaxer. Sometimes, when they want a perm, they'll ask for a curl. Ask clients if they want their hair straightened or chemically curled.

◆ Hair additions are often refered to as a *weave* in the African-American community. For the professional, weave refers to one possible attachment method.

◆ Teach clients a little about the words you use without overdoing it or making them feel foolish. If a client doesn't want to see red in his or her hair, show the client what ash looks like and ask if that is what he or she wants or if some warmth is desired. Then discuss what type of warmth (gold, red, etc.) and show examples with photos.

◆ Clients won't always tell the truth about previous services, especially when it comes to admitting to a professional that they performed chemical services at home. Typically, a long-time color client who "tried out" another salon or home color will be embarrassed to admit it. Watch for signs of discomfort in body language and let your hair analysis guide you. If you suspect a client is "holding out," don't turn it into a confrontation; discuss the service you feel your hair analysis permits.

LIFESTYLE CONSIDERATIONS

Some clients are accustomed to daily hair-care routines; others don't want to be bothered. Ask your clients how long they want to spend styling their hair each day. Styles that work with natural texture are often the easiest to maintain. If a client has fine, straight hair, or wants soft curl without daily roller setting, a perm might make the styling routine easier.

Services that require the most maintenance and upkeep are decolorized or bleached haircolors and relaxers, which require frequent conditioning and moisturizing.

If the client spends days in an office building that has dry air and little humidity, this, too, can affect a service decision. Such clients will have to condition their hair more frequently if they opt for a chemical service. If you live in a very humid climate, which causes hair to revert to its natural texture, you'll want to consider this as well.

Always determine what the client wants to get out of a particular style and whether or not the client's desires work well with his or her lifestyle and willingness to maintain a style. For instance, a client may ask for a curl because she wants versatility. However, a client who gets a two-step curl cannot blow dry, roller set and iron curl her hair daily without substantially weakening the curl. Make certain she realizes this prior to the service.

SKIN TONE AND EYE COLOR

Use skin tone and eye color to help guide haircolor decisions. In general, if you stay within two levels of the natural color, your results will be pleasing to the eye and natural-looking. If the client wants a dramatic change, determine whether her skin tone is blue or pink-based or yellow-based.

Yellow or gold-based skin tones look best with warm haircolors; blue or pink-based skin tones look best with cool or ashy colors. Hazel, green, topaz and warm brown eye colors look best with warm shades; blue, deep green, brown and almost-black eye colors are complemented by cool tones.

Some clients will want to break the rules or make dramatic statements in contrast, but these guidelines will help you and your client arrive at a decision. If a dark-haired client wants a much lighter haircolor, always explain the chemistry of the double process, the services with which it is incompatible and maintenance.

PERSONAL STYLE

If you greet your clients before they change into a robe, you'll get a better insight into their personal style. (Fig. 4.4) However, don't assume too much. A professional woman who must look conserva-

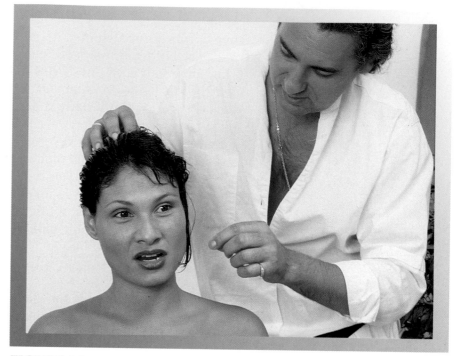

FIGURE 4.4
Talk with the client to determine her personal style. Photo: Steven Landis with direction from Vincent and Alfred Nardi of Nardi Salon, New York City, New York.

tive during the day may enjoy wearing more avant-garde fashions on her own time. Ask clients if they consider their personal style conservative, stylish, relaxed or extremely high-fashion.

Determine if the client wants a style that permits several variations for a professional look, a casual style, or one for special occasions. Such discussions can also lead to other service suggestions that involve the entire salon, for example, nail services and makeup that suit a client's personal image.

Some clients feel strongly about maintaining their natural hair texture. Always ask if your client wants a cut or style that allows him or her to avoid using chemicals. In all segments of the population, the "natural" approach to beauty is increasing in popularity. Do not view this as a trend; often it is a strong commitment that is tied to social, political or cultural beliefs.

ARRIVING AT A DECISION

All of the previous information will be used to arrive at a decision regarding the specific service, the type of product to use, processing times, maintenance, home care and future services. Before proceeding with any service, make certain you and your client have agreed upon the same look. Hair length and color decisions are particularly troublesome because there is the "hairdresser's inch" and the "client's inch," the warm haircolor and the brassy color. Often clients who don't want to see brass will say they don't want to see red or warm colors. You know that red can be warm or cool.

Reconfirm the requested length by showing the client in a mirror how short a cut will be or by using photos. Explain the "whys" of any suggestion you make. Don't tell clients they'll look "better" with short hair or bangs; tell them what these will do for their individual facial features.

If the hair's condition does not make relaxing, chemical curling or coloring safe, explain the consequences. Don't be so afraid you'll lose a client that you do something you know will be bad for the hair in the long run—especially if serious damage will result. If a service is contingent on conditioning, stress this point.

Whenever clients bring in photos, explain how the cut or style will look with their particular hair texture and density. If you keep your own clip book handy that shows several styles with different hair types, you can show a client just what you mean. When you cut coarse, thick, slightly wavy hair into long layers, the effect is very different than when you layer fine, thin, straight hair.

Once you and your client agree upon a service, let him or her know what else can be done during the next appointment with the look he or she will leave wearing. This gives the client something to think about between appointments and can possibly boost your income during the next visit.

THE "DIFFICULT" CLIENT

Arriving at a decision becomes most challenging with the "difficult" client. But is the client really difficult? Clients know their own hair because they live with it. Both men and women have strong opinions about what they like and dislike, in terms of personal style.

Never "push" a style on a client for your own ego gratification. If a client doesn't think he or she would look great in a look you suggest, give your reasons and let the client absorb the information for the next visit. Rhonda Shamburger, an cosmetology instructor in the Detroit area, offers these additional suggestions for dealing with the client who is a challenge:

◆ Most difficulties stem from a lack of communication. Explain the benefit to the client of anything you suggest.
◆ If a client isn't willing to make a change, often it's because he or she hasn't developed confidence in you. Work to build that confidence by using your well-rounded education to provide information, advice and service.

◆ Once you've completed the service, if the client insists on styling her own hair, allow her to do so. Use it as an opportunity to observe how the client prefers to wear her hair and how proficient she is at styling it. (Usually this occurs with female clients.)

◆ Minimize difficulties by presenting the "whys" of a service or service refusal in a professional manner. Use professional terminology and explain a little about products, chemistry and the hair.

◆ Be truthful, tactful and patient.

PRECAUTIONS

Once a stylist and client agree upon a service, most stylists get right to it. They routinely ignore the strand and patch tests, which are highly recommended in today's litigious society. Always test permanent haircolor for allergic reactions with a patch test; perform a strand test if henna or other color is present. If your hair analysis showed weakness, a high degree of porosity, breakage or any other contraindications to a chemical service, always perform a strand test first. Apply the relaxer, reducing agent and booster, or permanent wave solution on a small area at the nape and analyze the results before proceeding with a full service.

MAINTAINING CLIENT RECORDS

Develop a client record card that notes both overall hair texture and the texture around the hairline, natural curl configuration, porosity, tensile strength, overall condition and any other information that you'll want on file, such as evidence of mechanical damage. Note the results of patch tests and strand tests, as well.

While you're probably familiar with simple recordkeeping, keep in mind that with the chemical-service client, you'll want to perform a porosity test each time and compare it to your previous results. Since the population of over fifty-year-olds is increasing dramatically, you'll want to make a habit of recording prescription drugs your client is taking and their effect on services, if any.

Record cards provide vital technical information, but they're also useful for building a business. (Figs. 4.5, 4.6, 4.7) Develop a system that color-codes cards by the last time you saw the client, and you'll be able to regularly pull the cards of those who you haven't seen for a while and give them a call or send out a reminder notice. Ask if

PERMANENT WAVE RECORD

Name .... Tel. ....

Address .... City................... State ....

DESCRIPTION OF HAIR   Zip ....

Length	**Texture**	**Type**		**Porosity**

☐ short ☐ coarse ☐ normal ☐ very ☐ slightly
☐ medium ☐ medium ☐ resistant porous porous
☐ long ☐ fine ☐ tinted ☐ moderately ☐ resistant
☐ highlighted porous
☐ bleached ☐ normal

Condition

☐ very good ☐ good ☐ fair ☐ poor ☐ dry ☐ oily

Tinted with ....

Previously permed with...

TYPE OF PERM

☐ alkaline ☐ acid ☐ body wave ☐ other............................

No. of rods .... Lotion .... Strength ....

Results

☐ good ☐ poor ☐ too tight ☐ too loose

Date	Perm Used	Stylist	Date	Perm Used	Stylist
....	....	....	....	....	....
....	....	....	....	....	....
....	....	....	....	....	....

Other side of Record, continue with:

Date	Perm Used	Stylist	Date	Perm Used	Stylist

FIGURE 4.5
A permanent wave record.

they were unhappy with their last service or offer them an incentive to return— for example, a free conditioning treatment. If the salon in which you work is computerized, sending out reminder cards, birthday greetings and more is a matter of routine.

RELAXER RECORD

Name .... Tel. ....

Address .... City .... State .... Zip ....

DESCRIPTION OF HAIR

Form	Length	Texture		Porosity	
☐ wavy	☐ short	☐ coarse	☐ soft	☐ very porous	☐ less porous
☐ curly	☐ medium	☐ medium	☐ silky	☐ moderately	☐ least porous
☐ extra-curly	☐ long	☐ fine	☐ wiry	porous	☐ resistant
				☐ normal	

Condition

☐ virgin ☐ retouched ☐ dry ☐ oily ☐ lightened

Tinted with ....

Previously relaxed with (name of relaxer) ....

☐ Original sample of hair enclosed ☐ not enclosed

TYPE OF RELAXER OR STRAIGHTENER

☐ whole head ☐ retouch

☐ relaxer .... strength .... ☐ straightener .... strength ....

Results

☐ good ☐ poor ☐ sample of relaxed hair enclosed ☐ not enclosed

Date	Operator	Date	Operator
....	....	....	....
....	....	....	....
....	....	....	....

FIGURE 4.6
Recordkeeping for relaxing services.

FINDINGS AND INDICATIONS

The following at-a-glance chart lists potential findings of the analysis-based consultation and the services that they indicate. These indications are not hard and fast rules; other factors come into play as well.

HAIRCOLOR RECORD

Name _____ Tel. _____

Address _____ City _____

Patch Test: ☐ Negative ☐ Positive   Date _____

DESCRIPTION OF HAIR

Form	Length	Texture	Density	Porosity
☐ straight	☐ short	☐ coarse	☐ sparse	☐ very porous ☐ resistant
☐ wavy	☐ medium	☐ medium	☐ moderate	☐ porous ☐ very resistant
☐ curly	☐ long	☐ fine	☐ thick	☐ normal ☐ perm. waved

Natural hair color _____

	Level	Tone	Intensity
	(1-10)	(Warm, Cool, etc.)	(Mild, Medium, Strong)

Condition

☐ normal   ☐ dry   ☐ oily   ☐ faded   ☐ streaked (uneven)

% of gray _____   Distribution of gray _____

Previously lightened with_____for _____(time)

Previously tinted with_____for _____(time)

☐ original hair sample enclosed   ☐ original hair sample not enclosed

Desired hair color _____

	Level	Tone	Intensity
	(1-10)	(Warm, Cool, etc.)	(Mild, Medium, Strong)

CORRECTIVE TREATMENTS

Color filler used _____   Conditioning treatments with _____

HAIR TINTING PROCESS

whole head _____retouch inches (cm) _____shade desired _____

formula: (color/lightener) _____   application technique _____

Results: ☐ good   ☐ poor   ☐ too light   ☐ too dark   ☐ streaked

Comments: _____

_____

_____

_____

_____

Date	Operator	Price	Date	Operator	Price
_____	_____	_____	_____	_____	_____

FIGURE 4.7
A haircolor record.

FINDING	INDICATION
Scalp is sensitive.	Use a no-lye relaxer with a protective base creame; wrap two-step perm with conditioner as opposed to a curl booster; avoid bleach. (Or delay the service.)
Scalp is abraded.	Delay chemical service.
Scalp is inflexible and tight.	Do not perform hair addition services.
Oil/dandruff/scalp disease.	Refer to dermatologist.
Dry dandruff is present.	Treat with UV light; sterilize all tools.
Uneven curl configuration.	Use different timing or product strengths for different parts of the head when relaxing or perming.
Hair is extremely curly.	Use a medium-strength relaxer; two-step curl process.
Hair has an "S-shaped" curl.	Use a maximum strength relaxer; two-step curl process.
Hair is straight and coarse.	Use an alkaline perm and larger rods.(Using smaller rods will force the hair to shift too far from natural bonds.)
Hair is porous.	Use a gentler relaxer; condition prior to perming; use a filler prior to coloring.
Hair is overly porous.	Deep condition; delay relaxing and perming chemical services; use a filler prior to coloring hair.
Hair is fine and straight.	Use single-step perming process.
Medium texture, loose wave.	Use single-step perming process.
Hair shows evidence of breakage, tensile strength.	Trim the ends; if breakage is mid-shaft or lack of hair is weak, delay chemical services and hair addition services.
Henna traces on hair.	Perform a strand test prior to chemical services.
Metallic dyes traces on hair.	Remove prior to chemical services.
Permanent color traces on hair.	Use mild-strength relaxer, at least a week after the color was applied.
Sodium relaxer is on the hair.	Do not use a thio product.

FINDING	INDICATION
Thio product found on the hair.	Do not use a sodium or calcium product.
Hair is chemically straightened.	Test porosity, recondition and touch-up regrowth. (Or, press regrowth.)
Client wants relaxed hair.	No permanent haircolor the same day.
Wants low-maintenance style.	Cut hair to work with the natural curl configuration; suggest a perm or a bob for minimaldaily styling if hair is fine.
Dark-haired client wants to lighten hair two levels, plus.	Decolorize the hair or perform a double-process.
Client wants hair additions.	Double check scalp condition, flexibility.
Black client wants a perm.	Make certain she means a curl; discuss desired curl to make rod-size selection.
Client wants relaxer or curl and haircolor.	Discuss product limitations, waiting times.
Client wants a chemical service or haircut.	Call the client three days after the service to service or a haircut. ask him or her how the new style is working out.

the likelihood of cutting into the form. Generally, when you use clippers, the emphasis of the cut will be on the silhouette. (Fig. 5.3)

For extra control, some stylists use both hands to hold the clipper. When holding the clippers with one hand and the hair or a comb with the other, the more tension used, the more precise a line the clippers will create. This makes them an inappropriate choice for relaxed or fragile hair.

Clippers come with various blades, denoted in size by millimeters (mm). (Fig. 5.4) The 1 mm blade has the most closely spaced teeth, while the 5 mm blade has more widely spaced teeth. In general, the more widely the teeth are spaced, the more irregular the resulting line. When guiding the hair with your fingers, the 1 mm blade cuts closer, while the 5 mm blade automatically distances the hair to be cut from your guiding fingers.

Blades also come in straight, wedge and convex/concave shapes. The straight blade achieves the closest results, the wedge positions itself away from the scalp and the convex/concave blade curves gradually away from the head. The .000 (triple zero) blade is used for cutting necklines and the temple area. It is also used for free form cutting, to create a silhouette.

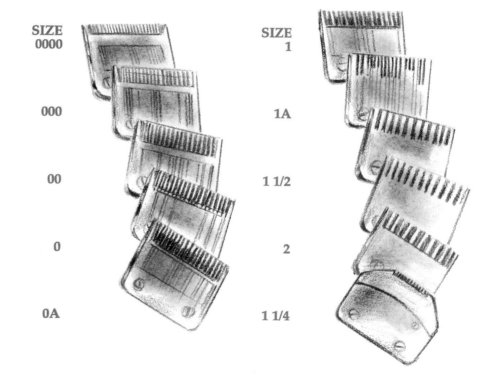

SIZE 0000 · 000 · 00 · 0 · 0A

SIZE 1 · 1A · 1 1/2 · 2 · 1 1/4

FIGURE 5.4
Blades for clippers come in various sizes. The 1-mm blade has the most closely spaced teeth.

USING RAZORS, THINNING SHEARS AND TEXTURIZING SHEARS

Razors are rarely used on hair that's more than moderately curly, except when cleaning up the nape area. (Fig. 5.5) Razors lightly taper the hair's ends and can be used to create beveled lines. With the razor, place your middle, ring and index fingers over the shank, then slightly close your hand, placing your thumb on the thumb grip or in the groove of the shank. Place your pinkie on the tang, or handle, and keep your wrist flexible. Generally, hair is razor cut when damp to avoid pulling the hair. Razors can be used to add slight mobility to the ends of fine, straight hair.

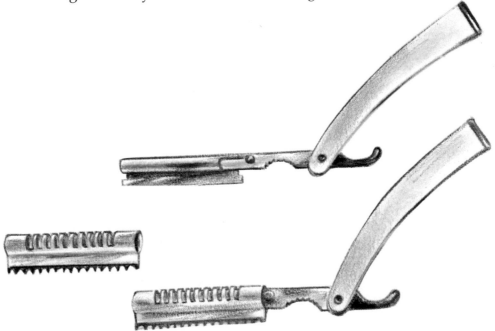

FIGURE 5.5
A razor.

At times you'll want to remove bulk from the hair by using thinning shears. These shears have one or both blades notched or serrated. (Fig. 5.6) The single-notched edge cuts more hair. To achieve even results, work very systematically. If hair is coarse or very curly, do not thin it extremely close to the scalp or the new growth will pop up through the top layer as the hair grows. Begin at least an inch-and-a-half from the scalp. If hair is fine and straight, you can begin as close as half-an-inch from the scalp because the hair will lie flatter on the head; however, it is unlikely you'll ever want to thin this type of hair. Thinning shears can also be used on a hair addition to make it look more natural.

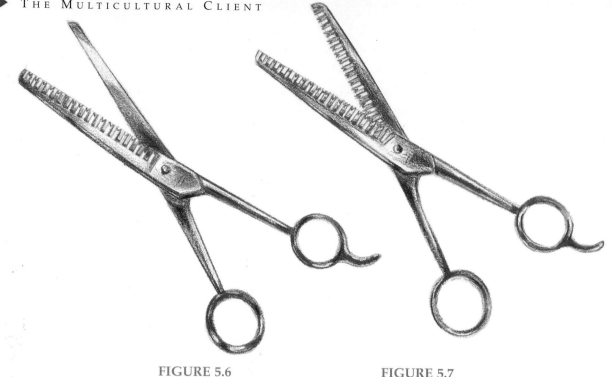

FIGURE 5.6
Thinning shears are used to remove bulk from the hair.

FIGURE 5.7
Texturizing shears are used for special-effect haircuts.

Texturizing shears come in a variety of shapes, with the blades spaced varying distances apart. (Fig. 5.7) These are used for special effects and should be used with caution on fine hair.

REVIEW: BLUNT CUTTING

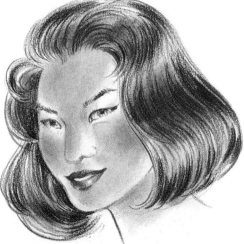

FIGURE 5.8
Blunt cutting. The basic bob.

To create a blunt cut or a basic bob, cut naturally straight hair damp or dry. Relaxed hair can be lightly dampened as you cut; very curly hair should be blown dry straight. If you choose to lightly dampen relaxed hair, keep in mind that when it dries it will contract. Even though it is relaxed, it will lengthen when wet, and dampening the hair is not advised if the hair is fragile.

1. Cut the hair as it naturally falls, using no elevation.
2. Begin at the nape and cut horizontal sections.
3. Complete the back, using the established guideline to determine the length.
4. Avoid using tension, particularly if hair is fragile.
5. When the back is completed, move to the side, bring down a subsection and match it to a portion of the previously cut back to create a new guideline.

6. Continue to bring down partings, cutting to the side guide line.

7. Repeat on the opposite side.

REVIEW: LAYERING

To create uniform layering, cut the hair at a ninety-degree angle. This maintains a rounded form. Hair can be layered when it is damp, if it is moderately curly to straight. (Keep in mind that it will stretch 40 to 50 percent of its length, especially if you use tension.) Each time you cut, use the previously cut parting as your guideline.

1. Use a five-section parting pattern and begin cutting at the front, establishing the length at the tip of the nose.

2. Continue working back, cutting the hair at a ninety-degree angle.

3. Complete the front-center section, move to the side and re-establish the guide, using the first parting that you cut in the center section as your guide.

4. Then work down toward the ear, holding the hair at a ninety-degree angle.

5. Complete both sides; then return to the crown and work toward the nape.

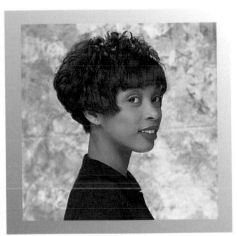

FIGURE 5.9
Uniform layering. The Halle Berry cut.

To create layers that progress from short to long, use a stationary guide to create a smooth progression. Hair is shortest at the front hairline and longest in back. Cut the hair damp if it is anywhere from straight to medium or moderately curly.

To create layers that progress in length, you generally begin cutting at the front and create a guide. Then hair is brought up to the guide as you work down the sides or toward the center back.

You can either use horizontal partings and bring the hair up to the guide as you work downward and backward, or use vertical partings and bring hair at the sides forward to a guide at the front hairline.

To alter the rate of increase, change the projection angle. The higher the projection angle, or the more the hair is projected out from the head, the greater the rate of increase.

If hair is too short to reach the initial guide, use mobile guidelines. For example, if you begin at the front hairline, once you reach the top of the head, make the last section that you cut your new guideline. Often you'll want to layer only a portion of the hair; for example, the front and top only.

When hair has a medium curl pattern or natural wave, it will naturally blend when layered and conceal minor errors more easily. Extremely straight, coarse hair will make errors the most evident.

REVIEW: GRADUATION

In the graduated cut, the hair lengths are actually shortest at the nape and longest on top, as they are with the solid cut. This can be seen when the hair is projected straight out from the head. However, with the graduated cut, the length progression is not as rapid; therefore the hair appears to stack up. The wedge is the best-known graduated cut.

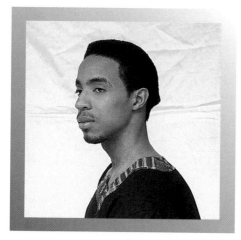

FIGURE 5.10
A graduated cut. The wedge.

1. Determine whether to cut hair damp or dry, based on the amount of natural curl. If hair is more than moderately curly, blow it dry straight prior to cutting, and keep contraction in mind when you establish the length. The curlier the hair, the less tension you should use when cutting.

2. Begin cutting in the back with no projection.

3. As you move up the head, lift the new parting and the previously cut one together and cut at a low projection angle.

4. Gradually lift each section higher as you cut it.

5. Remember, the higher you project the hair, the less distance the new section will travel to reach the guideline, and the shorter it will be once you cut it.

6. Keep your projection angle between zero and forty-five-degrees; do not lift hair any higher.

7. Cease projecting the hair at the point you want to end the graduation. Often only the perimeter of a cut is graduated, while the interior is solid.

REVIEW: SHAPING NATURAL CURL

To cut extremely curly hair, cut it dry and create a new silhouette.

1. Begin by using a wide-toothed comb or pick to comb the hair upward, extending it to its full length.

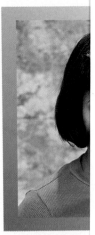

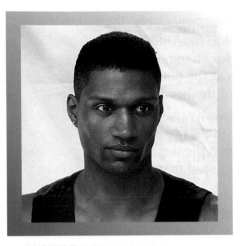

FIGURE 5.11
Shaping natural curl. The close fade.

FIGURE 5.1
A finished sty

2. Start at the crown and continue until the hair is evenly distributed around the head. Combing in a circular pattern helps avoid splits.
3. Begin cutting at the back or sides with the clipper.
4. Remove bulk first, then contour the design.

A wide variety of cuts are possible, from Afros to fades to high-top fades. These will be examined in detail in later chapters. Once the cut has been completed, the hair can be easily shaped with the hands.

REVIEW: PROJECTION ANGLES

When hair is projected out from the head, it creates an angle between the hair and the head shape. Always keep in mind that the head shape is a curved surface; therefore, when hair at the nape is held at ninety-degree angle, it will be held out horizontally, while hair held at a ninety-degree angle at the crown will be held up vertically.

When cutting, you usually start at the nape, establish a guide and work up the head, cutting horizontal sections. The higher you project the hair, the shorter the top sections will be. If you project the hair at a low angle and maintain that angle, the hair will get progressively longer as you work upward, because the hair will have to travel farther across the curve of the head to reach the guideline. While some stylists prefer to begin a cut at the side or the front, the laws of projection angles remain the same.

1. When hair falls straight down, it creates a solid line. The solid line is cut by using zero projection. The hair strands actually get longer from nape to crown, but fall to a single length.
2. When hair is projected to a forty-five-degree angle, it becomes graduated as longer hair "stacks up" on the ends of shorter sections below it.
3. When the hair is held at an angle that's higher than forty-five degrees, it becomes layered. That is, it gets progressively shorter from nape to crown.
4. When hair is held out at a ninety-degree angle, you can layer the entire head uniformly, by maintaining the projection angle throughout the entire cut and using a mobile guide. Each time

7. When layering hair that has wefts or hair additions, and layers are shortest in the interior and longest in the exterior, take care that you do not cut the top layers so short that the attachment site shows.

8. To blend natural hair with wefts, try bringing down sections and cutting them slightly longer than the previously cut section. This way, hair actually lengthens toward the interior, which is evident when all the hair is held out straight, at a ninety-degree angle from the head.

9. If you created synthetic or human hair braids which are to be cut later, pre-estimate the final length and heat seal the ends. Do not cut off the heat seal. You can pre-cut the hair fiber if you know how much length you will lose once they are braided. You can also tie the braids just above where you'll cut them, remove length and then heat seal them.

•••••
WI(

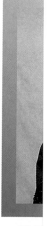

FIG
Hair
ume.

REVIEW OF CUTTING VARIOUS NATURAL CURL CONFIGURATIONS

Keep the following general rules in mind when cutting various hair types:

EXTREMELY CURLY

◆ Blow dry straight or chemically straighten prior to cutting.
◆ Or, pick the hair out to its full length prior to cutting.
◆ Cut the hair dry.
◆ Do not use tension.
◆ This hair type retracts the most as it dries: up to 50 percent.
◆ This hair is easily shaped with the clippers.
◆ This hair shows minute errors or "steps" when cut very close to the head.

MODERATELY CURLY OR S-SHAPED CURL

◆ Cut the hair damp.
◆ Use minimal or normal tension.
◆ Maintain a consistent level of moisture.
◆ If elasticity is good, hair stretches 40 to 50 percent its length when damp.
◆ Watch for uneven curl configuration.

SLIGHTLY WAVY

◆ Cut the hair damp.
◆ Use normal tension.
◆ This hair can be cut with a razor.

STRAIGHT, DENSE

◆ Cut the hair damp.
◆ Use fine partings when cutting with shears.
◆ You can use larger partings when cutting with the clippers.
◆ This hair shows minute errors the most easily.

STRAIGHT, MEDIUM TO FINE

◆ Cut the hair damp.
◆ When cutting with shears, you can use larger partings.
◆ If layering fine hair, lightly layer it dry to view your final results as you work. This technique helps you avoid over-layering fine hair.
◆ Lightly beveling the ends will help give this hair badly needed shape.

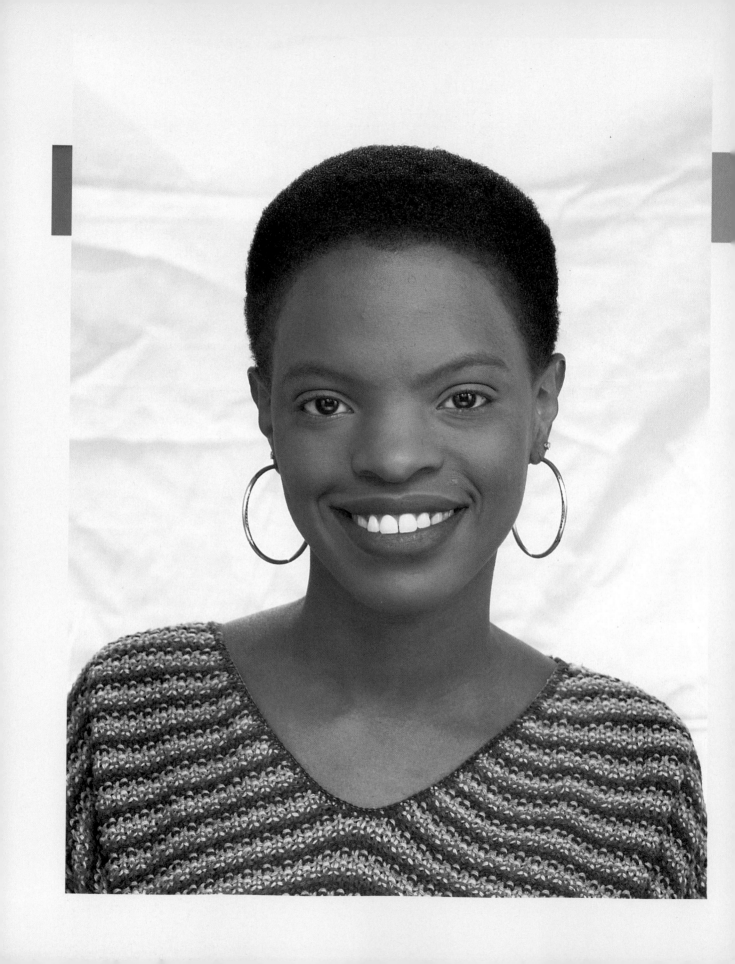

6

Advanced Women's Cuts

After reviewing the cutting basics, you should be able to combine different techniques to create a variety of styles. Hair can be cut at any number of angles, graduated up to a point to create a weight line and then completed with a blunt line, both layered and graduated in the same cut, or cut freeform into a wide variety of shapes if it is extremely curly.

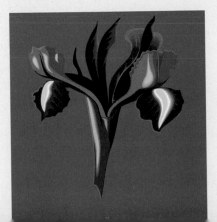

THE BASIC BOB

The foundation for the first cuts in this chapter is the basic bob, but the bob can take on a wide range of appearances, depending on which other techniques are applied. For example, angle your fingers downward at the sides (from front to back) and you can create a "diagonal back" line. Angle them upward and you can create a diagonal-forward moving line. Additionally, the nape can be cut into a *V*- or *U*-shape, or cut close to the head so that the solid bob line hangs over the close-cut nape. You can also create an asymmetrical bob by parting the hair on the side before beginning the cut. The two sides needn't be even.

When cutting a bob, keep the following tips in mind, which relate to hair texture and curl configuration:

◆ If hair is extremely curly, blow it dry straight first and keep the rules of contraction in mind. Extremely curly hair will contract 40 to 50 percent when it is dried. If hair is fragile and lacks elasticity, it will contract less.

◆ You can also relax the hair prior to cutting. Remember that if you then dampen the hair to cut it—or only partially dry the hair after relaxing it—the relaxed hair will contract 10 to 20 percent once it has completely dried.

◆ If hair has a medium-curl pattern, cut it damp and test its degree of contraction prior to cutting. Maintain uniform moisture. You can also partially air dry the hair to keep ends stable and avoid a "tug-of-war" with curl.

◆ If hair is permed with either a one- or two-step process, cut the hair after the perm has been completed. Cut permed hair damp, accounting for the fact that when dried, it will contract between 10 and 20 percent.

◆ If you're performing the cut with clippers, cut the hair dry.

◆ If hair is straight, cut it damp.

◆ If hair is coarse, take finer partings.

◆ In all cases, keep the client's head straight, unless you are designing a special nape shape by cutting against the skin. Then you can have the client lean forward to establish your initial line.

THE BOB AND ITS VARIATIONS

1. Relax the hair, dampen it or blow dry it straight, depending on the curl configuration and the client's desires. (Fig. 6.1)
2. Divide the hair into four sections. (Fig. 6.2)

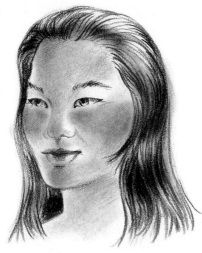

FIGURE 6.1
Blow dry the hair until it is straight and dry.

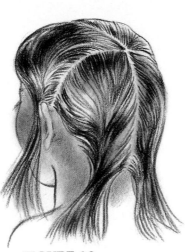

FIGURE 6.2
Four-section parting.

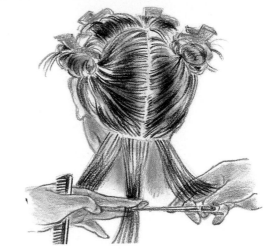

FIGURE 6.3
Use zero projection and cut the hair in a natural fall.

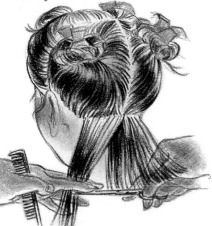

FIGURE 6.4
Cut hair to the established guide.

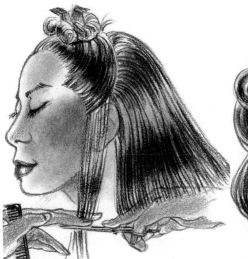

FIGURE 6.5
Hold the two sections together and cut.

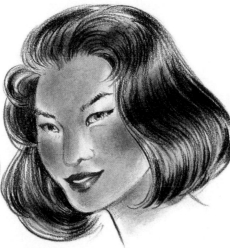

FIGURE 6.6
Finished style, "the bob."

3. Release a half-inch, horizontal parting at the nape and cut to the desired length, keeping contraction in mind. Use zero projection and cut the hair in natural fall; avoid applying tension if the hair is curly or has been physically or chemically relaxed. Continue cutting across the back to establish a guideline. (Fig. 6.3)

4. Bring down the next horizontal parting, adjusting the size of the parting to the hair type. The denser or curlier the hair, the finer the parting. Cut it to the established guide. (Fig. 6.4)

5. Continue working up the head, using horizontal partings and zero projection.

6. Next move to the side, release a horizontal parting and take a section of hair toward the back of the ear along with a section of hair from the previously cut guideline. Hold the two together and cut. (This extends the back guideline to the side.) Then continue cutting the side guideline. (Fig. 6.5)

7. Continue to cut horizontal partings, working up the side. Cut each parting to match the established guide.

8. Move to the opposite side and repeat steps 6 and 7. Be certain to use

minimal tension, particularly when you reach the partings that travel across the curve of the head. (Fig. 6.6)

THE DIAGONAL FORWARD OR DIAGONAL-BACK BOB

Generally, the bob that features a diagonal line is above the shoulder in length in order to show off the sharp, diagonal sideline. Pre-plan your back guideline with this angle in mind. If the hair is to move diagonally forward and be longest at the front, the back is generally cut shorter so that the side hair travels upward to join it. If the side is to move diagonally back, you'll want to establish a longer back guideline.

1. Cut the bob, following steps 1 through 5.

2. When you move to the side, take a portion of the back and a portion of the side and angle your fingers so that the two will blend, and then the side hair will continue along a diagonal. The steeper you angle your fingers, the sharper the line will be.

3. For a diagonal-forward line, look at the hair from the front and determine where you want the longer front to fall. Cut the hair along your angled fingers, to where the front and back sections will meet. Clean up the line and continue, using the new diagonal line as your side guideline.

4. For a diagonal-back line, angle your fingers so the shortest hair is around the face and the longest section meets the back. Cut this as your new side guideline. The side can blend with the back or remain unblended, depending on the desired look.

5. Either repeat the procedure on the opposite side, or for a variation, cut the opposite side straight. The latter is most often used with an asymmetrical cut. In the asymmetrical version, the hair is sectioned with a side part, the heavier side is cut along a diagonal-forward or diagonal-back angle and the lighter side is cut short and straight.

THE HALLE BERRY CUT

Some call it a layered bob, others call it a pixie, but most know this cut simply as the "Halle Berry" look, and it's requested by that name in salons all across the country. Charles Gregory of Charles Gregory Salon in Atlanta, Georgia, who is Ms. Berry's personal hairdresser, notes that the cut can be performed on hair that has been relaxed anywhere from 50 to 90 percent and is at least four-inches long at the top, crown and front. He shares his technique for creating the cut in the following steps:

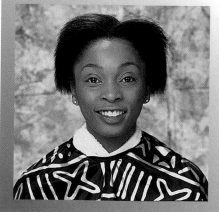

FIGURE 6.7
Before.

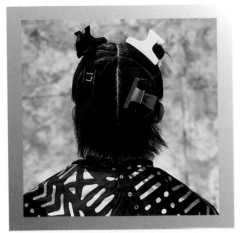

FIGURE 6.8
Five-section parting.

1. Section off the front from the back with an ear-to-ear parting that begins at the top center of one ear and moves across the top of the head, to the top center of the opposite ear. Then section off the nape with a horizontal parting that moves from the bottom of one ear lobe, straight across the occipital to the bottom of the opposite ear lobe. Finally, divide the top with a parting that moves from the center of the forehead, back to the horizontal part line at the occipital. This gives you a total of five sections. (Fig. 6.8)

2. Part off a one-inch section at the bottom of the nape with a horizontal parting. Cut it very close to the head, so the hair is approximately a quarter-inch long. This establishes your design line.

3. Now, move up the head and part off a quarter-inch, horizontal section. Cut the section so it is about three-and-a-half inches long. Comb all the hair at the nape up to the occipital, hold it out at a ninety-degree angle and cut it to the stationary guide. This will create length at the nape. (Fig. 6.9)

4. Next cut the top section into uniform layers. (The front should be parted from ear-to-ear, leaving a two-inch-wide fringe.) At the top center of the crown, part off a one-inch horizontal section or take a square section. Project it to a ninety-degree angle and cut straight across, so the hair is about three-and-a-half inches long. This becomes your guide for the crown. Leaving out the hairline, uniformly layer the interior to three-and-a-half inches by projecting each section to ninety-degrees and cutting to the guide. (Fig. 6.10)

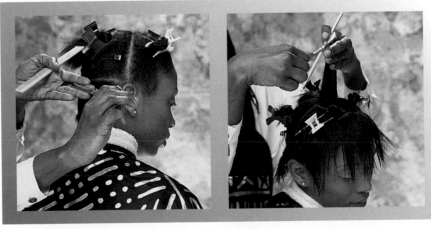

FIGURE 6.9
Hold hair at a ninety-degree angle and cut to the guide.

FIGURE 6.10
Uniformly layer to three-and-a-half inches.

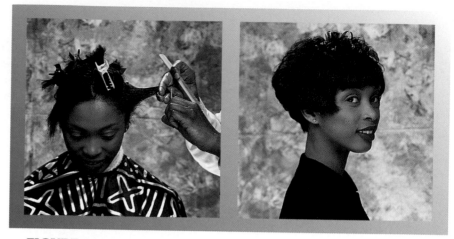

FIGURE 6.11
Project each section to ninety degrees and cut to the established guide.

FIGURE 6.12
Finished style, "the Halle Berry cut."

5. Work your way down to the sides and continue cutting to create uniform layers. Project each section to ninety degrees and use a mobile guide, so each section is about three-and-a-half inches long. (Fig. 6.11)

6. When the crown and sides are completed, comb the front section back to the guideline at the crown, project the front to ninety degrees and cut to the guide.

7. The finished cut can be styled with round brush, iron curled or set on small rollers.

THE SHORT, LAYERED CUT

The short, layered cut can be done on straight hair, extremely curly hair that has been relaxed or medium-curly hair that has been blown dry straight prior to cutting. Keep the rules of contraction in mind if you mechanically straighten hair that has medium curl. Eric Fisher of Eric Fisher Salon in Wichita, Kansas, and a member of the Joico International Team, recommends that you use a razor on straight or blown straight hair to get a softer feeling and avoid the look of freshly cut hair. Here is his technique for creating the look:

1. If the hair is medium curly, straighten it first, using a Denman brush and a blow dryer. Begin cutting at the nape, taking horizontal sections and cutting them so that an inch or two of length remains. This creates a longer, soft nape line.

2. Begin elevating the hair after the first three or four sections, depending on the desired look. Work up to the crown, elevating the hair slightly higher each time. When you reach the crown, hair should be elevated to forty-five degrees or slightly higher.

3. Next razor cut the sides to blend to the back nape line, cutting along a concave line. Cut the first section close to the head, using one-finger elevation.

4. Work up the sides to the top, progressively elevating the hair in the same manner as you did at the back. When you reach the top, hair is elevated slightly more than forty-five degrees.

5. Now comb the entire top and crown upward, hold the section straight up and remove any corners or points, using the razor.

6. Lastly, part off a half-inch curved section all around the face, bring it forward and razor cut to created a soft, rounded fringe. Bring down a second section and use the previously create fringe as a guide if you want a deeper, thicker fringe line. Finish the design by brushing through the hair and fingerstyling to enhance the soft, razor-cut texture.

THE SHORT AFRO

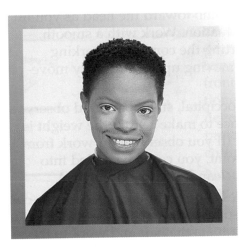

FIGURE 6.13
Before.

The short Afro for women is created by freeform cutting extremely curly hair, using a clipper and a jumbo comb. The hair is graduated from the perimeter up and is cut to work with the head shape. Eric Fisher of Eric Fisher Salon in Wichita, Kansas, and a member of the Joico International Team, uses the following technique, in which the hair is cut when it is dry:

1. First pick the hair out, using a jumbo comb with wide-set teeth. Observe its density closely—particularly if your client does not want much of the scalp to show through. Extremely curly hair gives the illusion that if it's cut close, you won't see the scalp, but density counts most when deciding how close to cut the hair. In this instance, based on the client's desires, only the first half-inch at the nape and sides is cut so close that some of the scalp shows through.

2. Begin at the nape and have the client lean forward with her chin resting on her chest. Cut the first quarter-inch, using a clipper-over-comb technique. Place the comb flat against the head. (Fig. 6.14)

beginning of graduation. Hair will be shortest at the nape and get longer as you move up the head.

8. Work from nape up to the horizontal guide, projecting hair at a forty-five-degree angle and cutting to the guide, until the nape is completed.

9. Now take a quarter-inch horizontal parting from the top of the ear to the center back. Comb the hair down, around the ear and onto the face. You can either leave the sideburns long or cut the hair into a *V*-shape. To create a *V*-shape, cut the hair in front of the ear on a diagonal line. Begin at the bottom and cut upward to the top of the ear.

10. Now take a horizontal parting that moves from the center of the back to just behind the ear. Project it to forty-five degrees and cut to blend the section to the nape.

LAYERED CUT FOR HAIR WITH ADDITIONS

When the client wants a layered look, hair additions or extensions are attached to hair that is at least shoulder length, which makes it possible to conceal the additions and layer the hair. (Additions can be used to add length or attached to shorter hair in braiding techniques, which will be discussed in Chapter 13). When layering hair with hair additions, the main principle to keep in mind is that you are primarily blending the hair; you are not taking the hair in horizontal subsections and cutting. The client wants the length and density of the hair wefts, so actual cutting is rarely performed.

Additionally, whether hair is straight or super curly, blending is done with a razor. If you use straight shears, the resulting effect will be unnatural, and any errors will stand out. The razor can be used on curly hair in this instance because very little of the natural hair is actually cut.

If you are going to remove length, pre-cut the client's hair before the additions are added. Then you can establish the length, which should be at least six inches, and blend the additions to the natural hair.

While detailed techniques for attaching hair additions will be explored in Chapter 12, the following technique includes steps for creating braided tracks and sewing in three to four hair additions or wefts for added volume.

Keiko Shino, an educator for Garland Drake International and a stylist at Avantage Salon in Tustin, California, shares the following tips and techniques for selecting, attaching and blending hair additions:

◆ Select a human hair or synthetic hair weft based on the client's desires. If she wants to style her hair straight or curly, suggest a human hair weft, which permits heat styling. Synthetic wefts should be ordered to match the client's natural curl configuration. They cannot be heat styled because they have a curl pattern that is "baked" into the hair; any heat implements will remove curl from synthetic hair.

◆ If the client's hair has a medium curl pattern and she wants to change her curl regularly with heat styling, blow dry the natural hair straight prior to adding the wefts and opt for human hair, which can be finished with heat styling.

◆ Always check the scalp's condition for red spots, tenderness or abrasions. Order the weft to match the client's natural color and texture, in the hair type desired. (Use a sample of her hair to do this.) It takes about a week for the additions to arrive, unless you have a wide range in stock. If you wait a week, recheck the client's scalp on the day of the service.

◆ Explain that shampooing, curling and styling will take longer, because these must be done more slowly and carefully, so as not to tug on or pull the wefts.

◆ On the day of the service, shampoo the hair and recheck the scalp. The wefts will be attached to wet hair in most cases. If the client has extremely curly hair, attach the wefts to dry hair. Keep in mind that as wet hair dries, it contracts and the tracks will get tighter.

◆ With the following method, create all the tracks first, then attach the wefts or hair additions. Perform blending with the razor last. If hair is very curly, layer it when it is dry—or layer it when it is damp, accounting for contraction. If the hair is medium curly, cut it damp; if it is straight, cut it when dry.

REVERSE LAYERED CUT

One popular cut that is layered throughout features the shortest lengths on top and the longest ones on the bottom. Richard Brown, a Detroit-area cosmetology instructor for Ms. Marion, Inc., developed a technique for creating the cut that is as simple as cutting by numbers. First the hair is divided into six subsections, then each subsection is cut in numerical order by bringing the hair within it up to a stationary guide. The fringe can be customized in any manner desired, and face-framing lengths can be added after the cut is completed, to further individualize the look.

1. To begin, comb the hair straight back, away from the face.

2. Divide the hair into six subsections. Beginning at the anterior, part a subsection that is approximately three-to-four-inches wide, which moves from the hairline to the crown. Next create two angled part lines, which extend from the lower corners of the first subsection to one inch behind the ears. Then extend the center section from the top of the crown to the nape hairline with two straight partings. Notice in the sketch that the center back subsection is labeled number 1; the subsection above it is labeled number 2; and subsections to either side of the center top are labeled 3 and 4. The lower-back side subsections, which were created with the angled part lines, are labeled numbers 5 and 6. (Fig. 6.19)

3. Starting at the top of subsection 1, take a half-inch to one-inch parting, comb the hair straight up to determine the top length and cut a stationary guide. (Remember, the top will be the shortest part of the cut.) Next cut all of subsection 1 by bringing partings up to the guide and cutting them.

4. Move to subsection 2. Take a half-inch to one-inch parting at the rear of the subsection, which includes a portion of your initial guide from subsection 1, and cut a guideline for subsection 2. Work toward the front hairline, bringing partings back to the guide and cutting, until all of subsection 2 is completed.

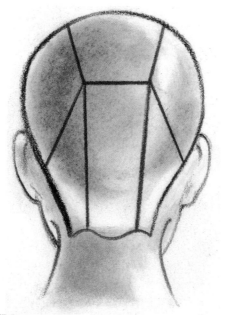

FIGURE 6.19
The hair, divided into six subsections.

5. Continue cutting the hair in the order the subsections are numbered until the cut is completed. Remember, with each subsection, take the initial guide along with a portion of the previously cut subsection. For instance, take the guide for subsection 3 right at the part line between subsections 2 and 3, then bring all partings in subsection 3 up to the guide and cut.

6. To complete the hair design, customize the fringe or create face-framing lengths as desired.

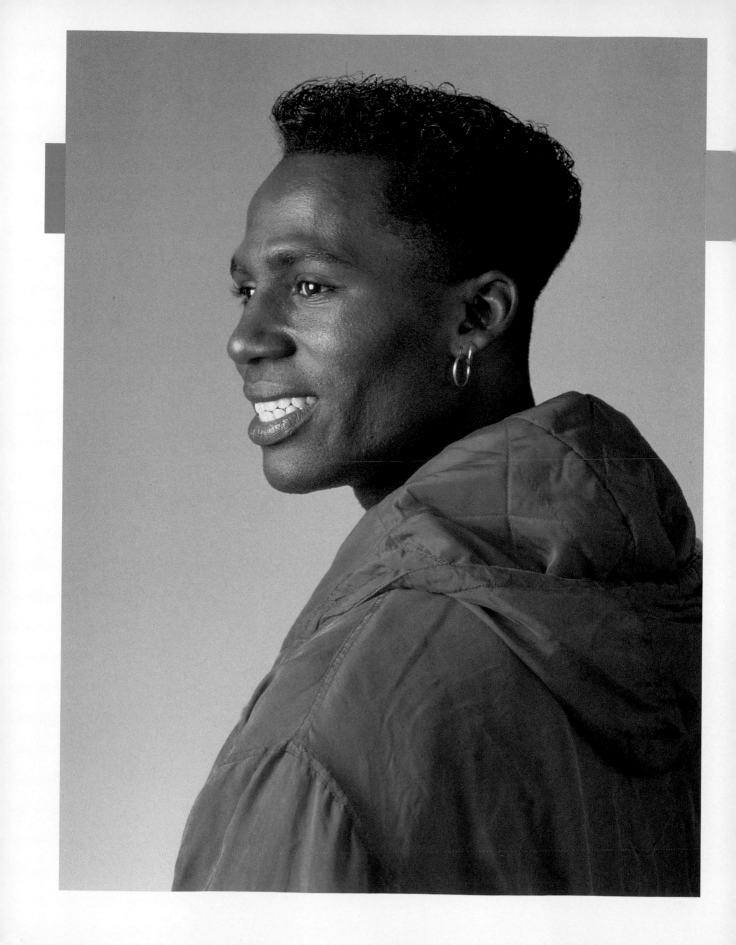

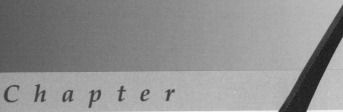

Advanced Men's Cuts

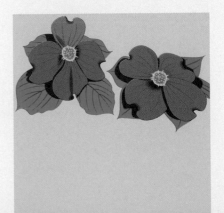

THE CLIPPER CUT, JUMBO AFRO

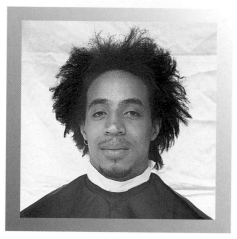

FIGURE 7.1
Before.

The jumbo 1970s' Afro is making a surprise resurgence, along with many other styles from the 1970s. For men who have extremely curly hair, the look is easily created by freeform clipper cutting a round silhouette after picking out the hair.

The style takes advantage of the hair's natural texture and its ability to hold any shape. Keep in mind that you are cutting a round shape on a rounded head-form. Use smooth, fluid movements as you cut the hair to follow the curve of the head.

1. Begin by picking the hair out to extend it to its full length. Work in small sections, beginning at the nape and working up to the sides and front.

2. First cut the nape line either straight across or into a slightly rounded shape, as desired. (Fig. 7.2) Then begin cutting from the nape up the back of the head.

3. Use smooth, even strokes to trim the ends of the hair, leaving maximum length. (Fig. 7.3) Follow the curve of the head, either working totally freeform or cutting clipper-over-comb. If you use a comb, choose a large wide-toothed comb and use it to hold the sections an even distance from the head as you rhythmically insert the comb, cut across it and move up and forward.

4. Work up the back of the head all the way to the front hairline, then move from side to side, continuing to cut the rounded shape. (Fig. 7.4) Use minimal pressure when cutting freeform.

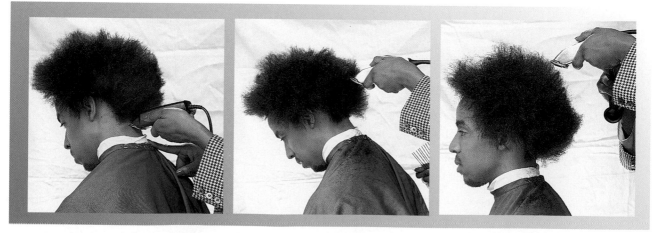

FIGURE 7.2
Cut the nape line.

FIGURE 7.3
Trim the ends of the hair.

FIGURE 7.4
Work up the back of the head to the front hairline.

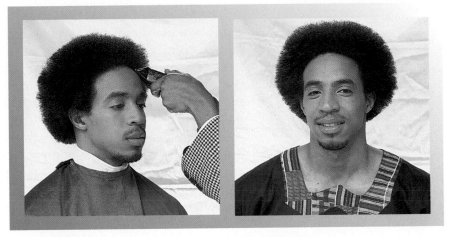

FIGURE 7.5
Using trimmer clippers, cut the front hairline and along the sides.

FIGURE 7.6
Finished style, "the clipper cut."

5. Move around the client as you work so that you can continuously observe the blade and make certain that the clipper cord does not touch the hair, if you are not using a cordless clipper. (A cordless clipper will make freeform cutting simpler, but some are not heavy-duty enough for cutting extremely curly hair in this fashion.)

6. Then move in front of the client, continuing to create a perfectly rounded form. When the rounded shape is completed, switch to the trimmer clippers. Detail the front by cutting straight across the front hairline and along the exterior form line at the sides. (Fig. 7.5) The trimmer helps you create sharp lines where desired. If you want the exterior rounded, use the regular clippers.

7. Shape the exterior form line with your hands and gently pat the rounded form into shape. Then use the clipper to clean up any stray hairs.

THE CLOSE FADE AND ITS VARIATIONS

The close fade, bald fade and high-top fade are all created on curly hair, using clipper-cutting techniques. According to John Young, an educator for the Wahl Corporation who resides in Pensacola, Florida, freeform clipper cutting permits stylists to transform super-curly hair into a wide variety of shapes because of the hair's nature and its ability to hold that shape. Similar styles can also be created on medium-curly hair, using a clipper-over-comb technique for control.

The foundation for a variety of the fade styles popular with men today is a close-cut sides and back, a blended area at the occipital, and customized front and top. To create the blend and remove any lines of demarcation, the clipper blade is opened or closed, based on the hair's density. For denser hair, the clipper blade is opened a bit more than halfway; for finer hair, it is opened slightly less than halfway.

The novice must become accustomed to the feel and cutting action of the clipper to become adept at freeform cutting. To avoid errors, maintain control of the clippers and practice until you are accustomed to the tool. Always cut against the hair's growth direction whenever you wish to achieve an extremely close cut. The only exception is when the client has a cowlick. These usually occur at the back of the crown or at the side of the front hairline. When a client has a cowlick, cut with the hair's growth direction to avoid nicking the scalp or possibly putting creating a gash.

What follows is Young's classic technique for the close fade, along with variations for the high-top fade, the bald fade and the ramp, which creates an angle at the top front. The steps given are for the client who has extremely curly hair.

THE CLOSE FADE

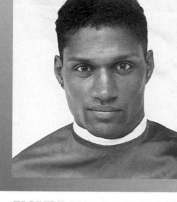

FIGURE 7.7
Before.

1. Set the clipper blade in the closed position (also called triple zero), to achieve the closest cut possible. The leverage will be in front. Start at the side, cutting upward (against growth direction), using a freeform technique. Cut around the ear and work up to just above the temple, cutting the hair extremely close to the head. (Fig. 7.8)

2. When you reach the area just above the temple, work toward the back, cutting from the perimeter up. (Fig. 7.9) Work with the curve of the head, cutting from the nape to just below the occipital.

3. Continue freeform cutting the hair extremely close to the head, as you work from the nape to the occipital and across the back of the head. When you reach the center back, work around the head to the opposite side. Then cut the side up to the same point just above the temple to which the previous side was cut. (Fig. 7.10)

4. When the back and sides are completed, adjust the clipper blade so it is one-quarter of the way open for fine hair or almost halfway open if the hair is dense. To create the fade effect, which removes any line of demarcation, begin cutting a quarter-inch horizontal section just above the area at the temple where you previously stopped cutting.

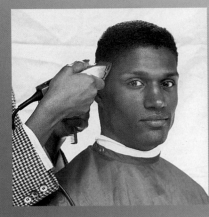

FIGURE 7.8
Cut around the ear and work up to just above the temple.

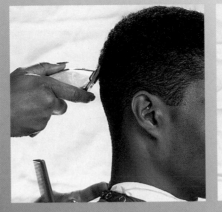

FIGURE 7.9
Work with the curve of the head. Cut from the nape to just below the occipital.

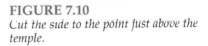

FIGURE 7.10
Cut the side to the point just above the temple.

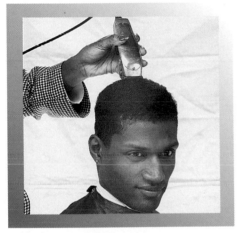

FIGURE 7.11
Work around the head, trimming any hair that protrudes outside the guide.

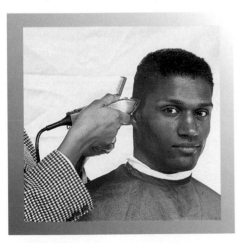

FIGURE 7.12
Return to the side and begin to graduate the hair.

5. Cut from one side, across the back of the head to the opposite side. Cut only the quarter-inch section as you move around the head.

6. Now open the blade another quarter (to three-quarters open if the hair is dense), and repeat the procedure. Work from right to left, across the back of the head to the opposite side, cutting a quarter-inch section just above the previously cut one.

7. When you reach the opposite side, repeat the procedure a third time. Open the blade all the way if the hair is dense and cut another quarter-inch section that moves from one side to the opposite, around the curve of the head.

8. Next place the #1 guard on the blade and position it halfway open. This allows you to cut the hair to a longer length. Repeat the procedure in step 5, cutting just above the previously cut section. This completes the blend.

9. When the blend is completed, remove the guard and close the clipper blade. Remove any hair that protrudes from the blend line, using a clipper-over-comb technique. Work all around the head, removing any hair that protrudes outside the guide. (Fig. 7.11)

10. Next move to the side and begin to graduate the hair. (Fig. 7.12) Work around the head until the desired degree of graduation is achieved, then complete the cut by uniformly layering the top and interior. If the

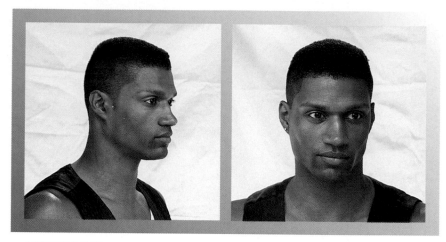

FIGURE 7.13
Finished style, "the close fade," side view.

FIGURE 7.14
Finished style.

hair is extremely curly, it is easy to graduate and uniformly cut the hair, using a freeform technique. If the hair has a medium curl configuration, use a clipper-over-comb technique.

11. To complete the cut, use the trimmer to define the front and side hairline.

THE HIGH-TOP FADE

1. Create the foundation for the fade, following steps 1 through 8 for the close fade.

2. When the blend is completed, pick the uncut hair out so that you can observe its full length.

3. Remove the guard from the clipper blade and begin cutting at the center top, at the crown. Determine how high you want the high-top to be and use a freeform technique to cut a straight line where the hair reaches that point. Cut from the top all the way to the front hairline.

4. Now cut either to the right or the left of the center section, using it as a length guide. When you reach the sides, create a square shape, using a freeform technique. Extremely curly hair makes cutting hair in this manner simple; if the hair is medium-curly, a flat top comb-over-clipper technique helps create the squared shape.

5. To complete the cut, use the trimmers to sharpen the squared edges, and define the front and side hairlines. Make certain that the top is uniform and that the edges are evened off.

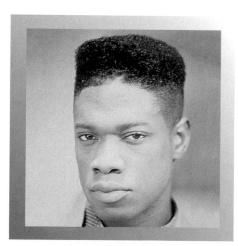

FIGURE 7.15
The high-top fade. Image: Aveda.

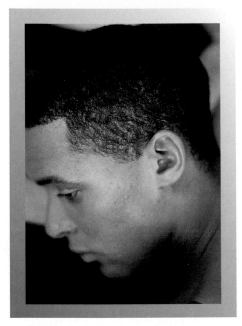

FIGURE 7.16
One version of a bald fade. Image: Aveda.

THE BALD FADE

1. Follow the procedure for the close fade, from steps 1 through 8. When the blend is completed, use the trimmers to cut the rest of the hair extremely close to the head, using a freeform technique.

2. Begin at the side, cutting against the hair's growth direction. Work up the side toward the center top, then move to the back and work up the head, from the occipital to the front hairline. Then continue to the opposite side.

3. Check the hair to make certain there is no line of demarcation. You may not need to create a blend line at all, since the idea is to cut the hair uniformly close.

THE RAMP

1. Cut the hair following steps 1 through 8 for the close fade. When the blend is completed, remove the guard from the clipper, close the blade and pick out the hair to its full, extended length. Remove any hair that extends beyond the guide.

2. Now move to the crown and point the clipper blade forward and out at an angle. Strive for a forty-five-degree angle and freeform cut the hair to the desired length, working from the crown to the front hairline.

3. Continue to cut the top at an angle, working out to the side you want highest first. Then return to the first section you cut and work toward the opposite side. The slant, or "ramp," can be positioned off center, as desired.

4. Now square off the sides and trim them to the blend line, if needed. Complete the cut by using the trimmer clippers to clean up the lines at the front and side hairline. If your edges are not sharp, reshape them with the trimmers.

Freeform Design Tip

The beginner who wants to cut freeform designs into the hair will find it easiest to cut out blocks where longer hair remains and introduce letters or shapes by cutting lines into the blocks.

THE WEDGE

The wedge is close-cut at the back and sides, but uses an exterior weight line to establish length almost immediately; therefore, most of the cut is not as close to the scalp as the fade. After the weight line is established, it is used to cut uniform lengths at the sides that increase toward the fringe (or bangs) and top. Essentially, it is a one-

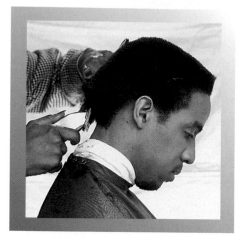

FIGURE 7.17
Use the clipper in an inverted fashion to build weight.

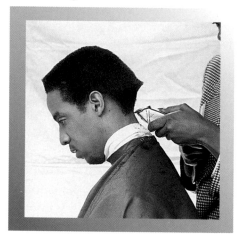

FIGURE 7.18
Reshape the bottom of the nape and the weight line.

length cut with graduation at the nape. On extremely curly hair, the cut is performed freeform, using a clipper on dry hair.

1. Begin at the nape by cutting the hair close, using the clipper. After cutting about a half-inch of hair very close, build weight toward the occipital by using the clipper in an inverted fashion. (Fig. 7.17) This creates a back weight line. Continue cutting with the clipper, cutting the hair to the length of the weight line.

2. Stop at the occipital and reshape the very bottom of the nape and the weight line just above it. (Fig. 7.18) Make the weight line as sharp as you desire.

3. Next move to the sides and cut the hair all around the ear in a curved line. (Fig. 7.19) Work from the front to the nape, cutting the hair very close to the head. After cutting the first half-inch very close, again invert the clipper to build a weight line.

4. Use the weight line as a guide to cut the next section; and continue in this manner, using each previously cut section as a guide. When freeform cutting, you do not have to pick up the guide; position the clipper an equal distance from the head each time. Stop when you reach the area above the temple, where you want the increase in length to begin.

5. Now angle the clipper to create an increase in length as you work to the top. (Fig. 7.20) Cut the hair so it will be longest at the top and the crown. When you

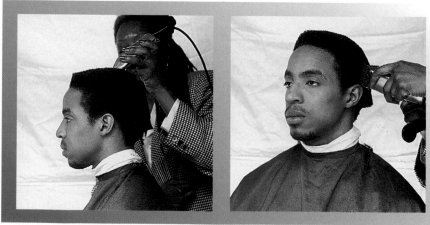

FIGURE 7.19
Cut the hair around the ears in a curved line. Then invert the clippers to build a weight line.

FIGURE 7.20
Angle the clippers as you work toward the top.

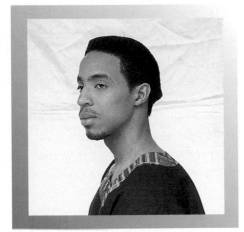

FIGURE 7.21
Finished style, "the wedge."

reach the center top, repeat the procedure on the opposite side.

6. Clean up the shape, then pick out the longer top and front to create a stronger, higher wedge, if desired.

THE MODIFIED WEDGE

The modified wedge has weight toward the back, as opposed to the front. To create it, when you reach step 5 for the wedge, establish the longest length at the crown and work forward, cutting sections closer to the head.

HEAD SHAVING

Head shaving is much more than a final option for the balding man who does not want a "comb-over." Today it is an accepted fashion statement, and numerous men with full heads of hair are choosing the style. Stylists who wish to offer the service should first check their state regulations. Many states do not allow cosmetologists who do not also have a barber's license to use razors. (The style cannot be created with clippers, since all the hair is completely removed.) Any stylist performing head shaving should follow sanitation regulations to the letter and keep informed of changes in those regulations. Always use a disposable razor blade or disposable razor.

Tommy Hicks, of Professional Results and Emages Hair Station, USA, in Houston, Texas, believes that salons should offer the service when regulations permit, rather than lose the business to the home market. Clients will attempt the service themselves, if profession options are not available. Here is his technique for today's hot new style trend: the bald look.

1. First examine the scalp for any contraindications to the service. If the scalp is abraded, has bumps or shows any evidence of a disorder, such as seborrhea, do not perform the service. If the scalp is in good condition, begin by removing excess length, using the clipper. Then, use the edger or the outliner to get as close to the scalp as possible. Shampoo the remaining hair and re-examine the scalp for any problem areas you may have missed.

2. Apply shaving foam or lather to the entire head, and apply a hot towel for two or three minutes. This softens the remaining stubble.

3. Begin shaving the back, working from the crown down to the nape. Hold the razor in a freehand position, use your opposite hand to pull the skin taut and shave with the growth direction of the hair to avoid excess irritation. Work from the crown to the nape in quick, short strokes, following the curve of the head. Keep in mind that because the head is curved, you should slightly overlap each section that you shaved, because the center of the razor is removing most of the hair.

4. Next have the client tip his head forward and continue shaving from the crown to the front hairline. Continue holding the skin taut with your free hand.

5. Complete the top section, then work down to the sides. When you reach the ear, hold the ear out of the way with your free hand and work carefully around it. Or have the client hold his ear down as you continue to work.

6. When all the hair is removed check to make certain you have not missed any areas. Then take a hot towel and remove all the excess lather. Apply witch hazel to the scalp, which is less stinging and will not clash with any cologne the client may be wearing. Follow the witch hazel with a cold towel for one or two minutes.

THE POMPADOUR

The pompadour gets its inspiration from the 1950s. In its modern version, it can be adapted for straight hair or super-curly hair. In this version, from Jon Rogers of The Place for Hair and Face in Los Angeles, hair is partially texturized to transform curl into waves, which support the pompadour style.

The technique shown is for extremely curly, virgin hair, which can be easily texturized into a wave pattern. If you want to texturize a medium or softer curl, extreme care is required to texturize the hair a small amount to achieve waves. Keep your eye on the hair, and check it frequently if it is less than extremely curly.

Thorough rinsing is extremely important. If you prematurely shampoo hair that has relaxer left on it, the shampoo could "slide" over the relaxer, and later, if the client perspires or it is humid outdoors, the relaxer could be reactivated. The nape area is the most neglected, because it is leaning against the sink, so make certain the nape is well rinsed and that no relaxer remains on the rim of the sink. When all the relaxer has been removed, the hair will not feel oily or smooth.

To create the classic pompadour shape, create a weight line at the sides, extend it around the head and use it as a guide to cut the back up to the crown. Once the front bangs are cut, the hair between the crown and the front can be individualized, depending on the client's facial shape, how round his head is or how defined he wants the final shape to be.

1. To transform extremely curly hair into waves, drape the client, put on gloves and apply a protective cream all along the hairline.

2. Examine the hair for an uneven curl pattern. Often curl is tightest at the crown. If curl is tighter in certain areas, apply the relaxer there first because it will take longer for the curl to release.

3. Begin applying medium-strength relaxer at the crown, using the back of the comb to evenly smooth on the product. Continue to the nape, which is also often resistant.

4. Continue applying the product at the sides, where softer curl occurs. (If hair is uniformly curly, do not wait the three to five minutes for resistant sections; apply product to the entire head at once.)

5. When the entire head has been covered with product, allow two to three minutes for the curl pattern to soften, then return to the crown and comb through it gently with a large-toothed comb. Do not force the comb through the hair; wait for the curl to release into waves.

6. Then move to the sides and comb through them. When you see the desired wave pattern, rinse the hair thoroughly and shampoo. Usually total processing time is fifteen to twenty minutes. To go from tight curl to a wave pattern requires approximately a 50 percent reduction in curl. However, each head of hair has its own "fingerprint" curl pattern and characteristics. Experience in both texturizing and in working with an individual's hair will give you the ability to predict texturizing results.

7. Part the hair into five subsections that separate the front from the back and the nape from the area above the occipital. (Fig. 7.22) First, part from ear-to-ear, across the top of the head, to section off the entire front. Then, divide the front into three equal-sized subsections by parting the center from the sides. (The part lines should be slightly above the eyebrow.) Next part the nape just below the occipital. Then observe the client's face to predetermine where you want the side weight line to occur. Base your decision on

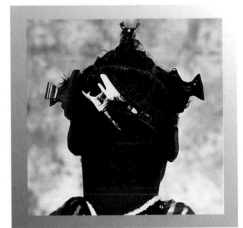

FIGURE 7.22
Five-section parting.

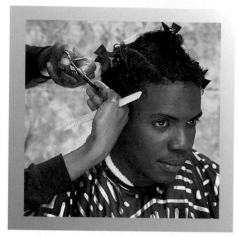

FIGURE 7.23
Direct the hair at a ninety-degree angle, slightly forward, and cut.

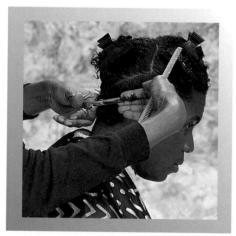

FIGURE 7.24
Angle the shears and blend sides to the

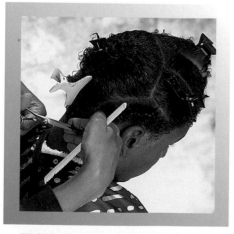

FIGURE 7.25
Angle fingers and cut the bottom of the nape.

esthetics, the client's desires and whether or not you want to create the illusion of either a slimmer or a wider face.

8. Begin the cut at the sides, which will be slightly longer than the close-cut back. For a precision cut, Rogers likes to start on the right side, work up to create a weight line, then repeat the procedure on the left side. He can then join the weight lines at the back, working around the head.

9. In front of the ear, cut the hair as close to the head as the bottom of the nape will be. Since this style will be worn back, cut the hair by first pulling it out at a ninety-degree angle and then directing it slightly forward, toward the face. (Fig. 7.23) With your fingers, create a diagonal back line so hair will be closest at the front and longest toward the back.

10. Next work up the head, slightly projecting the hair to build up to a weight line. Determine where the weight line will fall according to the client's facial shape. In some cases you may want the weight line to be placed just above the ear; in other cases, you'll want to create it at eye level. Once you have established the weight line, comb the remaining hair in this subsection straight down, and cut it to the guide all at once. (Remember, the center top remains sectioned off.) Repeat the procedure on the opposite side.

11. Then angle the shears to blend the side to the back. (Fig. 7.24) Cut from the side weight line to the nape, where hair will be the shortest. This continues the guide to the back, where it will be used to cut the entire nape area.

12. Take the continued guide, which occurs at the bottom of the ear, angle your fingers and cut the bottom of the nape to the guide line. (Fig. 7.25) Now cut half of the nape to the guide (for instance, the right side); then repeat the procedure on the opposite side. This way, you are working around the head, cutting half the nape from the right side to the center, then cutting the other half from the left side to the center. Stop when you reach the sectioned-off portion above the nape.

13. Now take horizontal sections and continue cutting them to the guide. Work up the head to the crown.

14. Next move to the front. Comb the bangs onto the forehead, part a half-inch parting and take a section of the

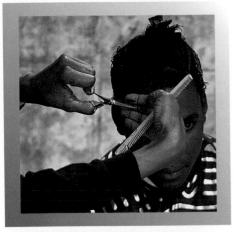

FIGURE 7.26
Cut the bangs, a half-section at a time.

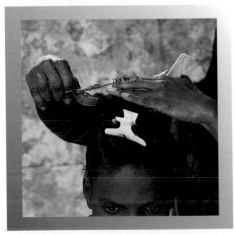

FIGURE 7.27
Project front subsection to a ninety-degree angle and cut.

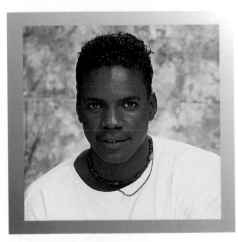

FIGURE 7.28
Finished style, "the pompadour."

weight line at the side with a portion of the bangs and cut the two together. Cut just to the center of the bangs, above the nose. (Fig. 7.26) Then take a section of the weight line on the opposite side and use it to cut the other half of the bangs. Check the bangs to make certain the line is even all the way across the front. This establishes your guide for the remaining center subsection. This subsection, which lies between the guide at the bangs (or fringe) and the guide at the crown can be individualized for the client.

15. To establish the long front of the classic pompadour, take a horizontal parting at the back of the subsection, project it to ninety degrees and cut to establish a guide. (Fig. 7.27) Next work forward, taking horizontal sections and bringing them back to the guide. After you have cut three to four partings, begin using a mobile guide. (Since the front length was established earlier, it will not reach a stationary guide.) Continue working forward, using a slowly advancing mobile guide until you reach the bangs. If you want a more rounded form, do not cut precisely to the guide; for a longer or heavier front, adjust the rate of increase and the length of the front guide.

16. When the center subsection is completed, check to make certain that no remaining hair overhangs the back weight line. Now remove weight to establish the final form. Most of the weight will be near the occipital, at the mid-back. After you have removed any excess weight, cross-check the entire cut by taking vertical partings where the hair was cut horizontally (and vice versa) and checking them.

17. For a variation, you can cut the center subsection by taking partings from the front and bringing them back to the guide at the crown. Begin at the crown and work forward, bringing each parting back. When you reach the front hairline, this section will be the longest, because it traveled farthest across the curve of the head to reach the guide.

18. To finish the style, you can set it in place with a freeze technique or apply mousse and dry the hair by either using a diffuser attachment or placing the client under heat lamps. The waves can be pushed close to the head with your hands, or the shape can be expanded by picking the hair out.

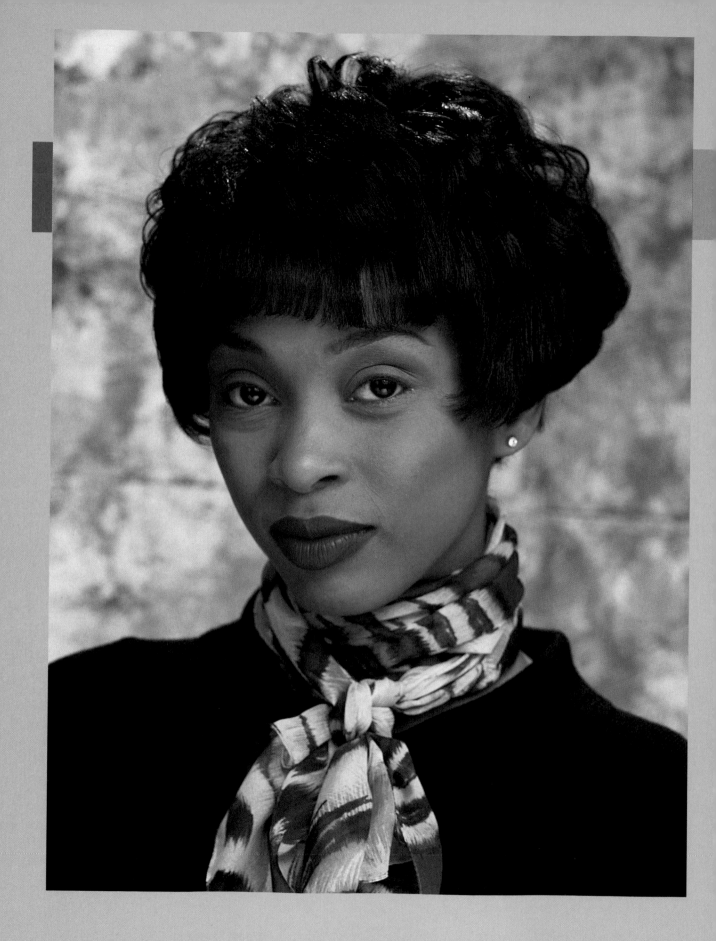

Styling Various Textures

All hair types can be straightened or curled with thermal styling and non-thermal techniques, such as roller setting. Many techniques can be used to temporarily alter the hair's natural texture. The primary ones are blow drying, pressing, iron curling, waving and roller setting. Short hair that has medium curl or less (natural or not) can also be molded or pin curled when it is wet, and dried under a dryer or allowed to air dry.

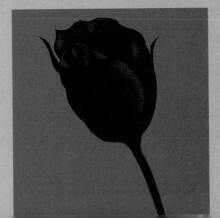

The weight of longer hair will pull waves downward, although long hair can be pin curled for soft curl. An overview of the primary techniques will give you the skills to alter any hair texture temporarily. Then you can mix and match various techniques to create a custom style.

BLOW DRYING

STRAIGHTENING

If you blow dry curly hair straight, it can then be cut into a bob, roller set or styled into a variety of looks. Either use a blow dryer with a comb attachment, a wide-toothed comb or a vent brush. Deep condition the hair first to protect it from moisture loss, and apply a blow drying lotion, which will help the comb glide through the hair with ease.

1. Part the hair into four sections, dividing it from ear-to-ear, across the top of the head, and from front to nape.
2. When the hair is wet, initially comb through the hair, gently working from the ends to the scalp to loosen the curl. Then begin drying to straighten the hair.
3. Begin blow drying a small subsection at the nape. Turn the comb or brush slightly to create tension as you dry, and use a heat concentrator attachment on the blow dryer. You can also use the comb attachment on your blow dryer.
4. Now work from the scalp to the ends, following the comb or vent brush with the blow dryer. Repeat the procedure as many times as necessary to dry the hair. Dry both the top and bottom of the subsections, using slight tension.
5. Continue through the four sections, drying the hair subsection by subsection. Take extra care at the hairline, where hair is more fragile.
6. Before re-curling the hair, check the scalp for any dampness. The hair should be completely dry before curling.

PRE-SETTING A STYLE FOR RELAXED HAIR

Hair that has been relaxed can be blow dried into the style in which it will be later set or curled. While this helps support the design and even allows you to set the hair using Velcro rollers, the following technique works best if the hair is going to be iron curled. The primary thing to remember is to remove excess moisture before beginning to style the hair by placing the client under the dryer. Then pre-blow dry the hair with the final, thermal-tool created style in mind.

1. To begin, apply a styling agent or leave-in conditioner. Then comb the hair. If the hair has soft curl, you can use an open brush. If it does not, separate hair with your fingers. Either place the client under a dryer or finger-separate the hair as you begin to remove the moisture, using the a warm setting on your blow dryer. Avoid hot settings, which can contribute to thermal damage.

2. Keep the dryer continuously moving as you remove moisture; when hair is 60 percent dry, divide the hair into four sections to begin styling the hair.

3. Begin at the nape, take a half-inch subsection and brush through it with a round brush. If you feel resistance, stop and begin again; avoid forcing the brush through or using excess tension. As it becomes easier to brush through the hair, you can switch to a Denman brush. Use it like a round brush, using the flat back of the brush to smooth the ends. This flat side acts like a pressing iron as you work.

4. Dry the hair in subsections with the finished style in mind. Keep the dryer moving continuously; do not concentrate the heat in any one area. Follow the direction of the brush with the blow dryer.

5. As the subsection dries, roll the hair around a round brush all the way to the scalp and finish drying, using a back-and-forth motion. Switch the heat setting to cool for a full minute or two before releasing the section.

6. If desired, clip the section in place. This makes iron curling simpler.

TIPS FOR ALL HAIR TYPES

When blow drying any type of hair, keep the following in mind:

◆ Always make certain the blow dryer is clean and that the air vents are free of lint. If the air intake is blocked, the dryer could short out.

◆ Use hot or warm settings to dry hair or remove moisture; use cool settings to "set" the curl in place.

◆ To avoid potential thermal damage, use the medium heat setting and keep the dryer moving continuously.

◆ Use thermal protectors, drying lotions and leave-in conditioners to protect the hair and make it easier to brush through.

◆ Avoid excess manual manipulation and extreme tension, particularly if hair is chemically treated.

- Hair that has been cold waved or permed using a two-step process cannot be blow dried daily without weakening the curl pattern.
- If hair is straight or fine, blow dry using a round brush to create volume.

PRESSING CURLY HAIR

Pressing is an alternative to chemically straightening hair, and it allows you to temporarily straighten extremely curly hair. The service works best on very curly, virgin hair and should not be performed on hair that is extremely dry or shows signs of excessive breakage. Generally the procedure is done with a pressing comb, although flat irons are still found in older salons and client's homes.

Pressing combs come in regular and electric styles. Regular combs can be heated on gas stoves or in electric heaters. Today most salons use electric heaters. In either case, the irons can be tested by touching them to either a tissue paper or end-wrapping paper. If the paper turns brown or becomes scorched, the comb is too hot to use on the hair and must be allowed to cool down.

Electric pressing combs simply plug into an outlet and are controlled by an on/off switch. A built-in thermostat maintains their temperature, which is a distinct advantage.

Neither type of pressing comb should ever be used at temperatures above 350 degrees. Fine hair will require less heat than coarse hair to straighten; if hair is damaged in any way, pressing combs and irons should always be used with extreme caution at lower temperatures.

To prepare the hair for pressing, shampoo and condition the hair, then blow it dry, using a comb attachment. Next apply pressing oil or cream to the clean, dry hair to protect it from heat damage, further condition it and add shine. Only products that are especially formulated to withstand the heat of a pressing comb should be used.

Most professionals recommend that you divide the hair into four sections prior to pressing and press the hair in subsections. The finer the hair, the larger the subsection you can press.

Keep these additional pointers in mind when pressing extremely curly hair:

- Never press damp hair. Prior to pressing, place the client under a hood dryer if there is any moisture present in the hair or on the scalp.
- The same rules apply to flatirons as to pressing combs.
- While some stylists recommend against it, chemically treated

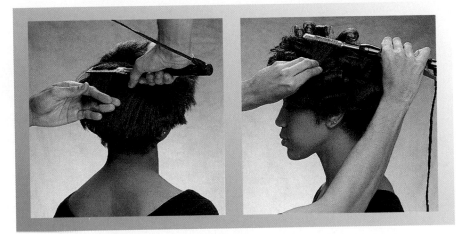

FIGURE 8.1
Wrap hair around comb. Comb will press against hair.

FIGURE 8.2
Touch up the hairline and nape.

hair can be pressed safely if you keep the hair in good condition with regular, professional conditioning treatments and use slightly lower temperatures than you would for virgin hair. However, there are usually alternatives to achieving the desired look that require less heat.

◆ Hair that has been permed using a two-step process cannot be frequently iron curled, pressed or blow dried without significantly weakening the curl pattern.

◆ If hair is extremely dry or shows evidence of breakage, treat the hair with a hot oil treatment and perform a "test press" before pressing all the hair.

◆ Remove tangles from the hair first by combing subsections without pressing hair against the back of the comb. (Use the ends of the teeth only.)

◆ The back of the comb or spine actually does the pressing; therefore insert the comb as close to the scalp as you can and quickly rotate the comb so that the hair wraps itself partly around the comb. The back of the comb should press against the hair. (Fig. 8.1)

◆ When using a regular pressing comb, return it to the stove or electric heater after you've completed each section and re-test it before proceeding. If the comb gets too hot, wrap a thick, damp cloth around it for five seconds.

◆ After all the hair has been pressed, touch up the hairline and the nape. (Fig. 8.2) If you are afraid of burning the scalp, insert a narrow metal comb between the scalp and the pressing comb until you gain proficiency. This protects the scalp from burns. (Don't use a plastic comb; it could melt from the heat of the pressing comb.)

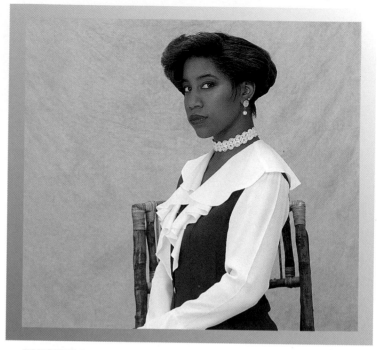

FIGURE 8.3
Finished style, "Hair pressing." Photo: Sally Russ for SalonOvations'
Beautiful Black Styles.

◆ A "root press" can be performed on the regrowth of relaxed hair between chemical retouches. Use extreme caution not to burn the scalp, and press the regrowth only.

HARD PRESSING VERSUS LIGHT PRESSING

Hair can be either hard pressed or light pressed. To light press the hair, use only as much heat as necessary to straighten the hair but maintain body. Two hundred to 250 degrees should be adequate. Hold the subsection away from the scalp with your index finger and thumb, then slowly draw the comb through the section. Press the hair against the back of the comb by turning your wrist after inserting the comb. Then reverse the comb and press the bottom of the subsection once. Move each pressed subsection out of the way as you progress from subsection to subsection.

To straighten extremely curly hair completely, use a hard press technique. The comb should be as hot as the hair will withstand. (Test a section at 300 degrees before progressing to 350 degrees.) Press the top twice before pressing the underside. Another technique is to reverse the comb so that the teeth face upward and press the back of the comb against the top surface of the subsection as you hold the ends. This allows you to "spot press" troublesome areas and remove the comb quickly. Once hair is hard pressed, it can be iron curled into any style.

IRON CURLING AFTER PRESSING

Curling irons also come in electric and stove- or oven-heated versions. Most hair can be curled using electric irons, which operate at lower temperatures than source-heated irons, which can get extremely hot. (Neither should be used at as high a temperature as a pressing comb is used; electric irons will not even reach those temperatures.) Stove-heated or Marcel irons are recommended for use on hair that has been hard pressed because higher temperatures are necessary to put curl back into the hair.

Whichever type of tool you use, test the curling iron by touching it to tissue paper before curling the hair. If the paper turns brown, the iron is too hot and should be cooled down by spritzing it with water or applying a thick, cool, wet towel for five seconds.

When extra hold is desired, hair can be curled using a curling iron, then the curls can be transferred to rollers or pin curls to cool down. Once hair cools, it will maintain its curl until the hair is exposed to moisture. When exposed to moisture, pressed hair will revert to its natural curl.

Moisture can be introduced by shampooing, by the client perspiring or walking outdoors into an extremely humid climate. If during the consultation the client indicates that he or she frequently prefers to wear the hair straight or slightly curled, relaxing the hair may be a better option—particularly if the client lives in a humid climate or exercises frequently.

Procedures for Iron Curling All Hair Types

Straight, slightly wavy, moderately curly and chemically relaxed hair can be iron curled to create a wide variety of styles. If the hair is relaxed and has been shampooed, blow it dry first, using the procedure described above. (Never iron curl wet hair.) Extremely curly hair can be blow dried or pressed straight prior to curling, for a temporary change in texture.

In all cases, pay extra attention to controlling the ends, and avoid touching the scalp with the iron as you create the finished style. Keep these additional tips in mind:

◆ Divide the hair into sections if you did not pre blow dry and clip sections in place. (Fig. 8.4)
◆ Begin by inserting the iron about a half-inch from the scalp. Hold it a few seconds to establish a base, then turn the iron to feed the ends into it. (Fig. 8.5) If you are afraid of burning a sensitive scalp, place a wide-toothed comb at the base of the section, between the iron and the scalp.
◆ To keep ends from crimping, smooth them carefully over the barrel. If hair is not extremely curly, you can

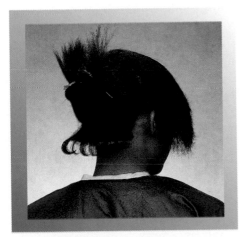

FIGURE 8.4
Divide the hair into sections and clip in place.

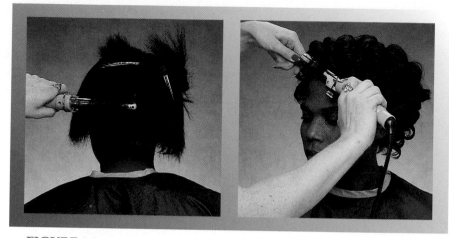

FIGURE 8.5
Insert the iron about a half-inch from scalp, and turn the iron to feed the ends into it.

FIGURE 8.6
Iron curl according to the predetermined style.

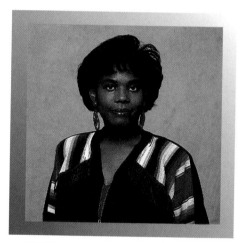

FIGURE 8.7
Finished style, "iron curling." Photo: Sally Russ for SalonOvations' Beautiful Black Styles.

also smooth the ends with your dampened fingers. This helps you to control the ends, but keep in mind that water will cause hair that is not naturally straight to revert.

◆ Hold the iron in place only as long as necessary and no longer than ten seconds. If the iron gets too hot as you continue to curl, spritz the barrel with water to cool it down, or apply a cool towel.

◆ If hair is short, establish the base and rotate the iron clockwise, opening and closing the lip rapidly to avoid creating creases in the hair with the lip or clamp of the iron. Continue to rotate the iron in a clockwise motion to guide the ends into the center of the curl.

◆ Iron curl hair with a predetermined design in mind. (Fig. 8.6)

THERMAL WAVING

Waves are a popular styling option. Hard-pressed hair can be waved with a hot, stove-heated iron; naturally straight hair can be waved with an electric curling iron. If hair is chemically relaxed, "test wave" it with an electric curling iron before opting for a hotter, stove-heated iron. The heat from the electric tool may be sufficient, and you'll be able to avoid excess heat exposure.

As stated previously, coarse hair can withstand more heat than fine hair, but always examine the hair's condition first and use a spritz-on thermal protector. If hair is dense, take finer sections.

PROCEDURES FOR WAVING HAIR

1. If the client has extremely curly hair and desires a temporary wave, press the hair first.

2. If the client has relaxed hair, shampoo the hair, apply a thermal protector or styling spritz, comb the hair and dry it, removing most of the moisture by placing the client under a warm dryer. When 60 percent of the moisture has been removed, blow dry the hair into the style in which it will be waved.

3. If the hair is naturally straight, remove all the moisture by using a blow dryer. Use the high heat setting until 50 percent of the moisture is removed; then switch to a low heat setting.

4. If the client has medium curl, blow dry the hair straight prior to waving so that the natural wave will not interfere with a deep Marcel wave. Or, if the hair type allows, use the slight natural wave to advantage.

5. When the hair is dry, it's ready to wave. Take a two-inch-wide section of hair, insert the iron close to the scalp with the lip on top, close it and position a comb just below the curling iron, inserting its teeth into the hair.

6. Draw the iron a quarter-inch to the right and the comb a quarter-inch to the left.

7. Holding the comb and iron in this position, roll the iron a quarter turn and hold the two in place for about ten seconds.

8. Now open the iron and re-insert it just below the wave you created.

9. Take the comb, insert it below the iron and repeat the procedure, waving the hair from top to ends.

10. Continue waving subsections until all the hair is waved. Pressed and relaxed hair will hold the style beautifully, and the surface can be lightly smoothed with a pomade to add shine. If hair is naturally straight and fine, add a touch of hairspray for extra hold.

ROLLER SETTING

Today there are more options than ever for roller setting. While traditional hot rollers work for any hair type, extremely curly hair must be blow dried or pressed first, meaning it will have been exposed to heat twice. For fragile, chemically treated or dry hair, Velcro rollers or moisture rollers may be a better choice than hot rollers. With Velcro rollers, the roller-set hair can be allowed to dry naturally or the client can be placed under a hood dryer.

No matter what type of rollers you choose, the type of curls you create relate to the base and the rollers' position in relation to it. There is no difference between roller setting naturally straight or curly hair, except that curly hair may require using more tension so that the hair closest to the scalp won't buckle. If hair is fine, you can take larger sections; if it is dense, take finer sections. However, keep in mind, that in either case, the smaller the section, the more curl you'll create—particularly with small-sized rollers.

BASE CONTROL

When you set hair, rollers sit on a base, which is the section that is created by making two partings. The partings can be vertical, horizontal or diagonal.

◆ For normal volume, the roller rests right in the center of the base, and the base is the same size diameter as the roller.
◆ If you want less volume, position the roller *half off-base,* in the lower half of the base. Or use partings that are larger than the roller's diameter and place the tool in the lower portion of the base. This is called *under-directed.*
◆ For extra volume, position the roller in the upper portion of the base and use a base that's larger than one diameter. This is called *over-directed.*

Remember, to achieve any type of volume, wrap the roller so that the stem is lifted, and turn the roller under. For indentation, the stem should lie flat and the curl should turn upward. These principles also apply to pin curling, iron curling and the use of any tool that sits on a base.

SETTING TIPS

Roller setting is one of the safest ways to style relaxed hair. For fullness, bricklay rollers. To create a combination of root lift or wave with end curl, first hold the roller horizontally and roll it up the strand about three revolutions. Then twist it into a vertical position and roll it end-over-end to the scalp. For three-dimensional waves, brush the hair out after setting and dry mold the hair in alternating directions. A hot blow comb can be used to accent the crest of the waves.

HEAT STYLING RELAXED HAIR SAFELY

Hair that has been chemically restructured with any form of hydroxide is considered to be relaxed. This hair requires special care and precautions when heat styling because heat styling can mask hair damage, creating an illusion of silkiness. The following information on safely heat styling relaxed hair comes from Rob Willis, a Soft Sheen educator who directs the Detroit-based "Future Legends" educational team.

Once, heat styling was primarily used to physically straighten virgin hair, creating a temporary texture change. Relaxed hair was wet set or waved because this was accepted as the healthiest way to style relaxed hair. As clients and stylists became more pressed for time, heat styling became the predominant form of styling relaxed hair, and today it is the fastest and most commonly used method— both in salons and at home. This is a change from past practices, and it puts hair at an increased risk of accumulative damage.

Today the stylist is faced with the question: Is the hair dry because of the relaxing service, excessive heat styling or both? The answer lies partially in the fact that if hair is not properly prepared to take heat, damage is almost assured. If hair is improperly processed, it will have a frizzy or "shattered" appearance, which heat styling conceals. The client will think the hair is in healthy condition, when in reality, it is damaged.

Compounding the issue is the fact that stylists and most clients use a hairdressing oil and hairspray to finish the style. These products make the hairstyle look better and last longer, but once the hair is shampooed and build-up is removed, damage becomes evident. Over time, the combination of relaxers, heat and styling products that conceal hair damage add up to a serious threat to healthy hair.

PROPER PREPARATION OF RELAXED HAIR

Relaxed hair should be consistently treated with a proper balance of moisture and protein conditioners. These help the hair to retain a natural, healthy balance and a soft-to-the-touch feel.

Prior to any application of heat to relaxed hair, shampoo it with a conditioning shampoo that promotes cleansing without stripping the hair of its natural oils. Then towel blot the excess water from the hair and apply a moisturizing protein treatment. Put a plastic cap over the hair, and place the client under a warm dryer for fifteen minutes. After the prescribed time, rinse the hair thoroughly and apply a styling lotion, distributing it evenly throughout the hair. You can now mold the hair into the desired finished style and place the client back under the dryer until the hair is at least 90 percent dry. For optimum hair health, do not blow dry the hair when it is wet.

Once the hair is 90 percent dry, you can safely blow dry it and use heat styling tools. If the hair needs to be straighter, apply a moisturizing cream to the hair and blow it dry into the desired style. Simple olive oil is an excellent hair dressing, because it penetrates the hair shaft, locking in shine and moisture without a heavy, greasy feeling. Do not use heavy spritzes; these are finishing tools, not hair preparatory tools.

If you wish to iron curl the hair or use hot rollers, do so after the hair has been completely blow dried. For styling coarse hair, the curling iron should always be tempered and clean, and maintained at a temperature of about 225 degrees. Test the iron or hot rollers first to make certain they are not excessively hot. If if heat styling tools are used at temperatures over 225 degrees, the hair could actually melt.

While other blow drying techniques presented in this chapter do not require that 90 percent of the moisture be removed first, the above method is the absolute safest for prepping relaxed hair prior to any heat styling. Any time hair health is an issue, opt for the safest techniques.

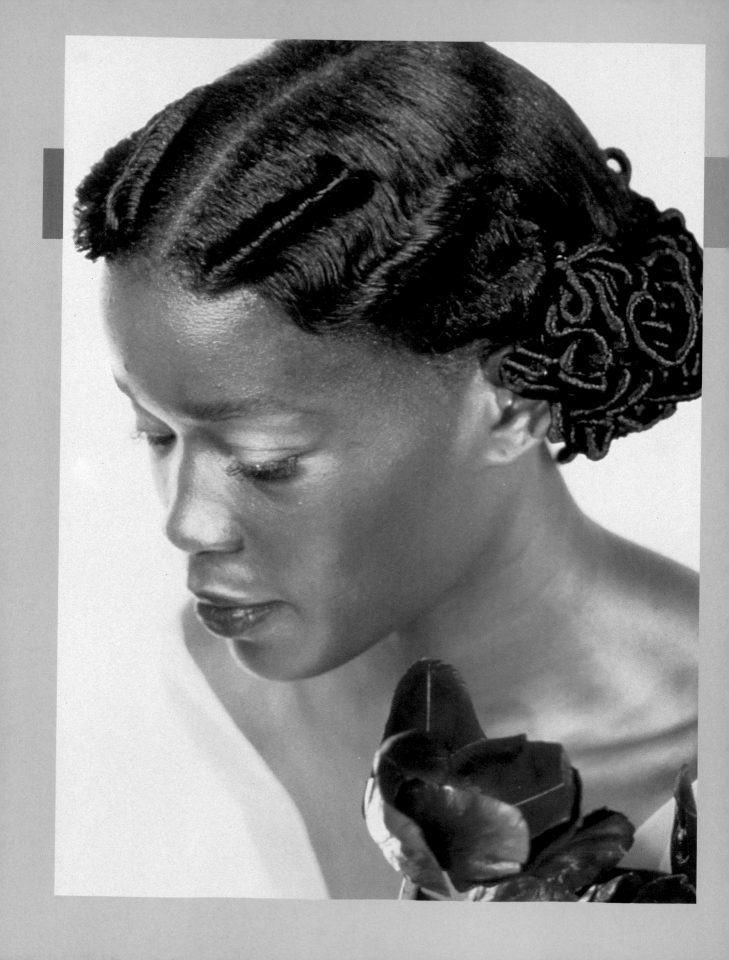

Advanced Styling Techniques

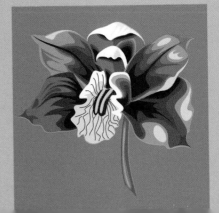

THE WRAP

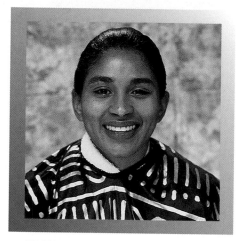

FIGURE 9.1
Before.

One of the newest styles, the wrap, is created by applying wrapping lotion to relaxed hair and "wrapping" the lengths in a single direction around the head. The hair design can be left as is, close to the head, or combed out. Wrapped styles with extra volume can also be created by using rollers that are wrapped in a single direction at the top.(Hold the rollers in place with a net while the hair dries.) Jon Rogers, of the Place for Hair and Face in Los Angeles, provides this traditional wrap technique, for a style that lasts a long as a week. It's perfect for active clients because it makes hair more manageable and gives it added movement. When applying the wrapping solution, keep in mind that the less solution you use, the faster the hair will dry.

The product used for wrapping should be one specifically formulated to create the wrap style. It is a liquid gel that can be slightly watered down, if desired.

1. If the hair has regrowth, perform a relaxer touch-up first. Then mix the wrapping solution with water to achieve the desired consistency. Apply the wrapping solution to the hair, combing it through from scalp to ends. Make certain the product is evenly distributed. Then begin wrapping at the crown, using a rattail comb to comb the hair in a counterclockwise direction. (Fig. 9.2)

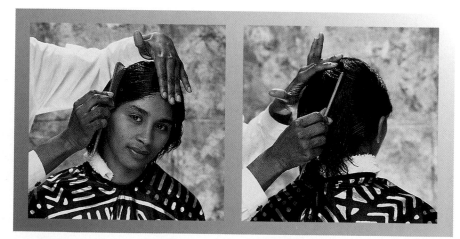

FIGURE 9.2
Begin wrapping hair at the crown. Wrap in a counterclockwise direction.

FIGURE 9.3
Comb and smooth small diagonal sections toward the front in a counterclockwise direction. Then work down the head.

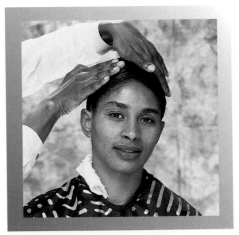

FIGURE 9.4
Smooth the front hairline.

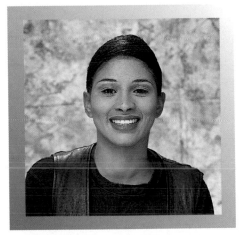

FIGURE 9.5
Finished style, "the wrap."

2. Continue combing and smoothing the hair in a counterclockwise direction, working from the crown forward and across the front.

3. Complete the hair from the crown to the front first. Strive to achieve a cone-shaped effect.

4. Then move to the side that will move back, and work down it, continuing to comb and smooth the hair to follow the curve of the head.

5. When the side is completed, move to the opposite side and comb and smooth the hair forward.

6. Now work toward the back, taking small, diagonal sections, combing and smoothing them toward the front in a counterclockwise motion. Work down the head, combing the hair up and across the curve of the head so that it "wraps" around the head shape in a circular pattern. (Fig. 9.3)

7. Check the hair to make certain the top is smooth. Re-smooth any hair at the crown that does not create a fluid, cone shape.

8. Now smooth the front hairline and check the entire style to make certain the hair is completely smooth and that it moves around the head evenly. (Fig. 9.4) Smooth all the hair with your hands, and put the client under a dryer until the hair is completely dry.

9. You can either leave the style as is or comb out the wrapped lengths. Comb out the hair with a large-toothed comb, and style the ends with a flatiron or a curling iron, if desired.

FINGERWAVES

Hair sculpting skills allow you to create a variety of classic designs, including fingerwaves and pencil-thin waves. Waves can be wet-molded into any type of hair, although straight and relaxed hair hold them best. Waves can also be dry-molded into hair that has been roller set with the direction of the waves in mind.

Balmer Galindez, of Salon D 'n' B in New York City, has a diverse clientele and staff that includes Americans of Asian, African and

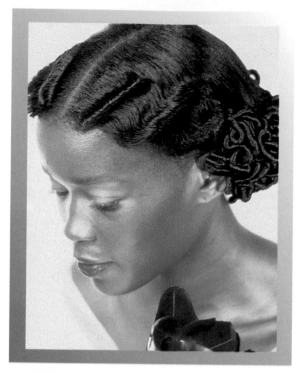

FIGURE 9.6
Finished style, "fingerwaves." Hair: Dennis Cooper;
Makeup: Kimberly Olson; Photo: Peter Harasty.

European origin, whose hair ranges from super-curly to straight. According to him, although waves can be created with almost any haircut, the ideal foundation for them is a short cut that's about two-and-a-half inches long, tight at the nape and layered throughout. The layers permit you to add wispy details around the perimeter.

If extremely curly hair is not relaxed, it can be blown straight prior to fingerwaving. If hair is relaxed, begin with the hair damp and apply gel. If hair has a moderate curl pattern, create the waves when the hair is wet to the point of saturation and use a bit more gel that you would for straight or relaxed hair. If hair is straight or has been mechanically straightened, begin with damp hair and apply gel. (Avoid heavy gels; a lightweight gel works best if polishers will be used to finish the style.)

Then use this precise fingerwaving technique from Salon D 'n' B:

1. Apply a quarter-sized amount of gel, beginning at the top crown. So you do not get excess gel in any one area, comb it through the hair by combing the top portion, then dividing the hair in half at mid-back and combing in each direction. Next apply gel at the front and repeat the procedure. By parting the hair and combing in two directions, you avoid concentrating the gel at the hairline. Use more or less gel as needed, depending on the hair's density.

2. Next "read" the front hairline by pushing the hair forward slightly. Determine the natural movement, or if there are cowlicks that must be accommodated. The movement of the hairline will determine whether you use a side, diagonal or center part. In this example, a center part will be used.

3. Comb the hair down from the part and begin molding at the part line. Create the open end of the wave first. Keeping the hair flat to the head, comb it into a "C" or half-moon shape that moves smoothly from the part line on a diagonal toward the face. For larger wave, make a large "C"; for smaller waves, create a small, tight movement. The crest of the wave occurs where the "C" shape ends.

4. To create the crest, hold your index finger in place at the bottom of the curve. Then use the comb to push in the crest from

front to back. Push up a small amount of hair each time, working back in quarter-inch to half-inch increments. This allows you to smoothly push up the hair directly below your index finger. Continue pushing in the crest all the way to the back of your finger.

5. To create the second half of the wave, lift your index finger, and position your middle finger at the top of the crest and your index finger below it, so that you are "pinching" the crest between your two fingers. The next crest will be created directly below the index finger. (If you want a wave that is wider than finger-width, you do not have to "pinch" the crest tightly. Move your index finger down a bit and hold the hair firmly in place by pushing against the head.)

6. Now push in the crest below your index finger by pushing the hair upward in small increments. Work from front to back. The two crests complete one wave.

7. Continue working down the head, creating waves in the same manner until you run out of hair.

8. Repeat the procedure for creating waves on the opposite side of the head. Strive for symmetrical waves by aligning the first "C" shape with the one of the opposite side of the part. (If your part is asymmetrical, you may want to create smaller waves on the opposite side.) Work down the head, aligning the waves.

9. When the front is completed, move to the back and connect the waves. Using the crest line as a guide, comb the hair from the crown into a "C" shape that ends right where the first side crest does. Then move to the opposite back side and connect that side wave to the back by creating another wave. The two back waves should connect to the sides and to one another.

10. Continue working down the back, creating waves that connect. You can either move side-to-side and down, or complete one back side and then the other, as preferred. Working from side-to-side allows you to easily connect the waves all the way around the head.

11. When you reach the nape, if the wave you just completed moves from left to right, end by creating a large "C" shape from the left. This closes off the nape. You can also mold the nape close to the head or comb it straight down.

12. Allow the hair to completely dry under a hood dryer, then dry-mold the lines of the waves by combing them in place, using the same technique that you used to create the waves. Complete the style by gently smoothing a shiner over the surface of the hair, using your palms.

FINGERWAVING PERMED HAIR

Hair that is permed or has a natural medium curl is the most difficult to fingerwave because you are fighting an existing curl pattern. To fingerwave this type of hair, air dry it first, then apply gel or mousse to the comb and comb through the hair several times to distribute the product and create the first "C" shape. Push or force the crest into place quickly, hold it in position and blow dry it in place. When the crest is set in place, continue down the head, repeating the waving technique.

....

THE FREEZE

In 1989 Joyce Williams of Kansas City, Missouri, created a totally new style for men, women and children called "the freeze." The style came about when Williams over-processed her husband's hair and used gel to push waves back into the bone-straight hair. After two days, she notice that the gel flaked, so she hired a chemist to develop products that would hold hair in place without flaking or discoloring hair and used them to create a style that would actually last two weeks, or until the hair is shampooed.

According to Williams, while the freeze is ideal for hair that's been 80 percent relaxed, the techniques used to create the style can be adapted for naturally straight hair or hair that has a medium-curl pattern. Hair can be short or shoulder-length, dense or fine. In fact, the style makes fine hair look denser by camouflaging thinning areas at the crown. The only firm requirement for creating the look is that you use products especially developed to create the freeze. Regular styling or molding gel will not "freeze" the style in place, and they will flake if used with this technique. The spray gel used should be one that is designed to work with the freeze system.

Here is Williams's own technique for creating the freeze, along with her tips for adjusting the procedure based on hair type and the client's desires.

1. If the client has extremely curly hair, relax it prior to creating the freeze. After processing is completed, thoroughly rinse out the relaxing product, stabilize and shampoo. If the client has a two-step, curly perm; natural, medium curl; or straight hair, shampoo the hair and lightly towel dry.

2. Next apply the leave-in conditioner. Use a leave-in conditioner that's formulated to work with the freeze gel.

3. Saturate the hair well with an alcohol-free setting lotion, comb it through, then follow with the freeze gel. Comb to

evenly distribute the product along the hair shaft.

4. Make certain that the hair is combed smoothly. If it is long, comb the hair up, piling the longer lengths on top of the head. Then re-smooth the hair all around the perimeter, working toward the top of the head.

5. Begin pushing in waves, using two combs. One should be a rattail comb with a long end. Begin at the front hairline. (If you prefer, you can begin at the nape or at the sides.) Comb through the hair from the hairline back. How far back you comb will determine the width of the wave; how far you push the wave forward will determine its height.

6. Next push the comb forward to form a wave. Place the end of the rattail comb behind the teeth of the first comb, right at the back of the wave, and hold it in place. Remove the first comb and use it to comb the hair behind the wave back, then push the comb forward again to create a second wave. If the hair is straight, use a clip to hold the waves in place. If hair is medium curly or has a two-step perm, observe the wave to determine if it requires a clip to hold it in place or not.

7. Continue the two-comb technique, working from the perimeter inward. After you have established three or four waves at your starting point, move to another part of the head, such as the sides or nape. The idea is to work in a circular pattern around the head, moving upward and inward as you create waves. Stop when a small circle of hair remains at the top of the head. If the hair is very short, you can complete the entire head, using the two-comb technique. You can also "design" the waves so that the side waves are more horizontal or waves are smaller at the sides and nape, and larger and deeper in front.

8. Now sculpt the hair that remains at the top into the desired shape. If the hair is long, gently comb through it, pull all the hair up in a single section and fold it down in a zig-zag pattern, the way you would fold a long strip of ribbon. Use the end of the rattail comb to hold each section as you fold the hair back and forth. The remaining hair can also be pin curled in a circular pattern or rolled into a single roll.

9. Now spray all the hair with the spray gel, which seals the cuticle and traps the product in the hair. Place the client under the dryer until the hair is completely dry. Usually this takes at least thirty minutes.

10. The hairstyle can either be left as is or lifted and picked into a fuller or higher style. If your client chooses the latter, mist the area you want to lift with the spray gel and use a metal pick to

lift the hair into the desired shape. Individualize the look to the client's tastes and facial shape.

The style can now be maintained for up to two weeks, using hair polish and spritz. Show your client how to use the products to lightly smooth his or her style each morning. That is all that's required, and sleeping with a hairnet is not necessary—the style holds that strongly. If the client opts to wear the style un-lifted for a week and wants to lift the style into a new shape for the final week, sell the spray gel as a take-home product and instruct the client to mist the hair and lift it with a pick to create a lifted style. Since the style can only be achieved by a hairstylist, it's a good idea to rebook the next appointment before your client leaves. At the next booking, rinse and shampoo the hair, massaging the scalp as you work. Since hair normally sheds fifty to eighty strands a day, after two weeks it is normal to see that amount of shedding multiplied by fourteen (days). After shampooing, you can condition the hair, apply the leave-in conditioner and create an entirely new freeze style.

HIGH-STANDING CRIMPS

The freeze technique can also be used to create high-standing crimps and many other designs that are limited only by your hair sculpting skills. High crimps are created using the basic freeze technique, except all the hair is combed to the center top and smoothed around the perimeter prior to sculpting. Then the hair that is piled on top is sculpted using a fingerwaving method or the two-comb fingerwave technique, which is performed by pushing in waves as you work from the base of the hair upward. Sharp, crimped waves can be created all over or in front only.

After the freeze style is dried in place, the hair on top can be misted with the spray gel and pulled out even higher.

THE FRENCH TWIST

The French twist is easy to create and can transform relaxed hair into an evening style in a half-hour appointment. To make the top roll fuller and higher, use a weft of human or synthetic hair that is close to the client's natural color and is about an inch in diameter. Cut it to the desired length by placing it two to three inches above the client's nape and bringing it across the top of her head to the crown.

The style can also be created for clients who have extremely curly hair by blow drying the hair straight. If your client has a medium curl pattern, you can create the style using her natural curl, but it won't look as smooth. Let esthetics and the final effect be your

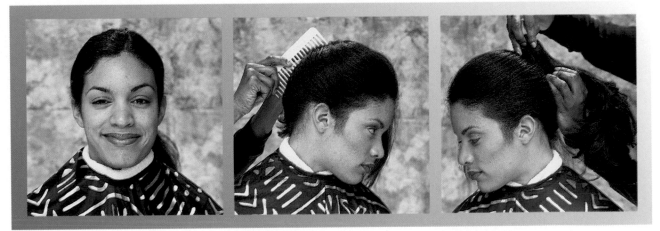

FIGURE 9.7
Before.

FIGURE 9.8
Comb all the hair to one side.

FIGURE 9.9
Twist the hair and tuck it under the artificial weft.

guide. The only times the style is not advisable are when the client's hair is too fine to conceal the hairpiece or the client's hair is shorter than two to three inches.

1. To begin, comb all the hair to one side with a large-toothed comb. (Fig. 9.8) Smooth the shorter side up and make certain the hair is combed across the back smoothly.

2. Hold the hair in place and position the artificial hair about two inches above the nape, draping it toward the crown. Then begin twisting the hair and tucking it under the artificial weft. (Fig. 9.9)

3. Smooth the sides up as you hold the hair and the weft in place with the opposite hand. Then continue to twist the hair and tuck it under as you move toward the crown. (Fig. 9.10) Use

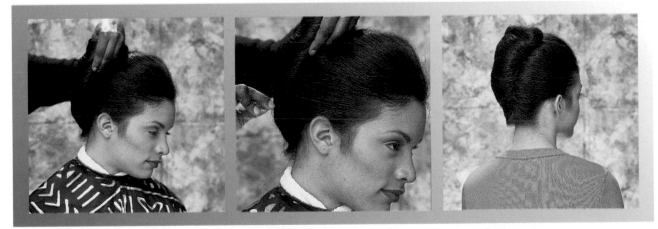

FIGURE 9.10
Using tension, twist and tuck the ends under.

FIGURE 9.11
Secure the hair with bobby pins.

FIGURE 9.12
Finished style, "the French twist."

tension to twist the hair and tuck the ends under and recomb the sides with a comb if necessary as you move forward.

4. When you reach the top of the head, tuck the ends underneath. Secure the hair all along the roll with bobby pins. (Fig. 9.11) If the client has bangs, incorporate them into the style by either backcombing them to further conceal the front section or gelling then back.

THE HALO OR HAIR ROLL

This simple style can be created in a half-hour by blow drying the hair straight and taking a few minutes to roll it up evenly. With some variations, it will work for any hair texture, creating a different effect with each. Hair should be at least six-inches long to create the roll design; if hair is shorter you can create a variation, using a headband.

1. If the hair is extremely curly, begin by blow drying the hair straight. If it is naturally straight, comb through all the lengths so they are smooth.

2. For long hair, have the client bend forward at the waist and comb all the hair from the neck forward.

3. Take the hair just behind the ear, while the client's head is still bent forward and begin rolling it under, working toward the middle forehead.

4. Continue rolling, using your thumb and fingers to create a thick roll. At the center forehead, if desired, create a slightly looser roll that will move forward. Continue rolling toward the opposite ear, keeping the hair above the roll smooth.

5. At the back, take all the ends and roll them under, securing them in place with bobby pins. Smooth the roll and spray lightly.

6. For short hair that is not overly fine in texture, have the client hold her head upright and distribute the hair evenly all around the head, combing it from the center top. Make certain there is enough hair on the forehead.

7. Place a headband on top of the hair, sliding it down so the top of the head looks like a dome. Keep the headband above the forehead.

8. Next, carefully tuck the ends of the hair underneath the headband all around the head. Make certain the hair is smooth and

even so that it conceals all of the headband. This style works very well for extremely curly hair that has been blown straight.

· ·

THE QUICK CURL

Mid-length hair that has been relaxed can be quickly styled into sideswept curls for a day-to-evening transformation. The same look can be created on naturally straight hair by iron curling the hair without blow drying it first.

The following technique, from Fantasia, emphasizes proper preparation and protection of relaxed hair prior to heat styling:

1. Begin by shampooing the relaxed hair and conditioning it with a reconstructor especially formulated for relaxed hair. Then apply a gel moisturizer/activator evenly throughout the hair to add moisture prior to heat styling and to make the hair easier to comb. Next apply a your preferred styling aid, such as a grow complex, to the roots and scalp only. This further protects them from thermal damage.

2. Blow dry the hair, beginning at the nape. Take horizontal sections and dry the hair, turning it under. At the front, direct the hair off the face as you blow dry. Drying the hair in the direction it will ultimately be styled reinforces the style, helping it to last longer.

3. After blow drying is completed, apply a quarter-sized amount of oil moisturizer to the hair to repair, strengthen and add shine. Rub the product between your palms, then work it into the hair with your hands. This further protects relaxed hair from thermal damage.

4. Divide the hair into four sections and spray it with a heat styling mist to further protect it from heat damage. Then begin iron curling the hair on the side to which it will be swept. Work from the side to the top, bringing the hair from the opposite side over when you reach the center of the head. Use an iron that has a large-diameter barrel to create larger curls; if desired, switch to a smaller size when you reach the hair on the opposite side. This creates tighter curl on top and more volume underneath.

5. When you reach the opposite side, smooth the hair close to the head and touch up the ends. Place the curls forward or back as desired and clip in place with concealed bobby pins as needed. Comb the back smoothly over to the side and lightly mist with hairspray.

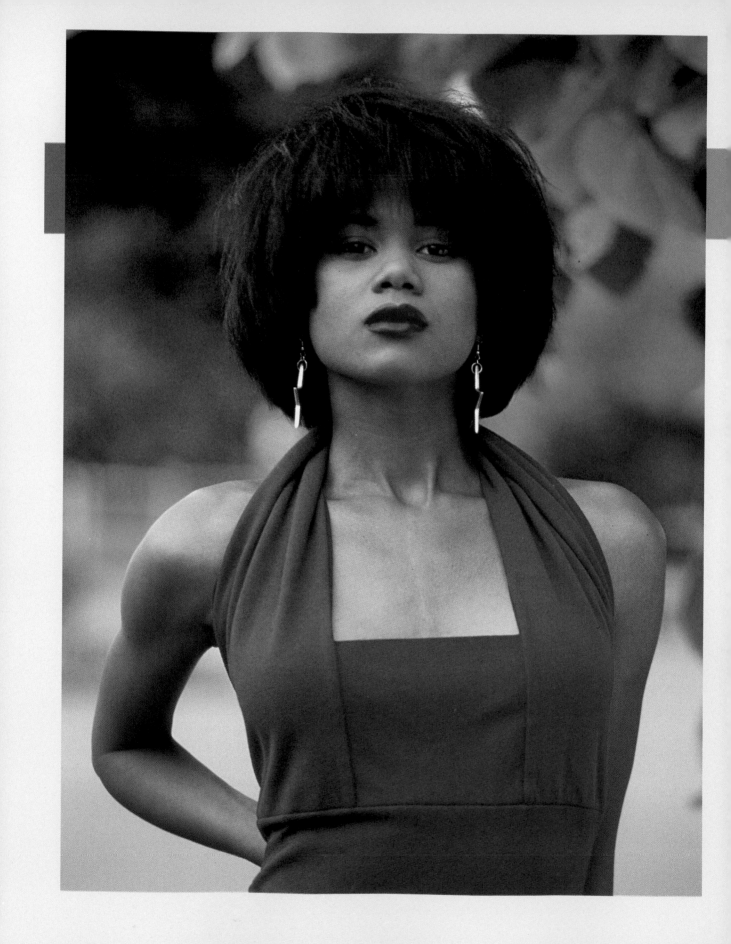

10

Relaxing and Texturizing Techniques

Relaxers are essentially hair straighteners; the terms are interchangeable. Chemical relaxing and texturizing services reduce the amount of curl in hair to varying degrees, depending on the existing curl pattern, the product used and the timing of the service.

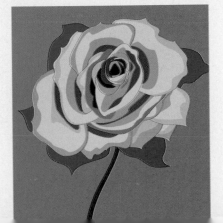

There are two basic types of relaxers: **sodium hydroxide,** which does not allow pre-shampooing, and **ammonium thioglycolate,** which does allow pre-shampooing, if needed. These two products are absolutely incompatible; therefore, one should never be used on hair that has been exposed to the other.

Traditionally, the action of relaxers has been explained as the breaking of the cross bonds (sulfur and hydrogen), which are then realigned and rehardened into the new, straightened formation. Some say that relaxers actually erode the hair's cuticle; others say that thio-based products transform cystine bonds into other types of bonds. All relaxers swell the cuticle and soften the hair.

Thick, coarse, resistant hair takes the longest time to relax; fine, porous or color-treated hair relaxes the fastest. Gray hair is often resistant, but is not necessarily so. Avoid making assumptions about any hair type; always perform a porosity test prior to relaxing or texturizing.

TYPES OF RELAXERS

Sodium hydroxide relaxers range from mild to super strength, depending on the percentage of sodium hydroxide and the pH of the product. In general, the more sodium hydroxide in the product and the higher the pH, the quicker the action of the relaxer—and the greater the potential for hair damage. Super-strength relaxers should be used on extremely resistant hair only. (Try a medium-strength product first, during the patch test.)

A sodium hydroxide relaxer is best for the client who wants to keep the hair straight. These lye-based treatments are not reversible and can only be grown out. After relaxing, the hair can be styled into various curl configurations through roller setting, iron curling, fingerwaving and other techniques, just like naturally straight hair can.

Lye-based products are stronger than thio-based products, but are less drying to the hair.

Ammonium thioglycolate products are somewhat milder and are generally used prior to a two-step perm. They may also be a better choice for fine or color-treated hair, which will relax rather quickly, or for somewhat sensitive scalps. Their action is similar to sodium hydroxide, although the final bonding chemistry is considered to be somewhat different. (Theoretically, this is why hair that is relaxed with a lye or hydroxide-family product cannot be chemically curled; the resulting lanthionine bond cannot be transformed into the type of bond required for curl.) If a client wants the hair straightened or texturized and may want a curl at a later date, a thio relaxer is an excellent choice because it is compatible with a thio-based perm. Since thioglycolate is drying to the hair, moisturizing after a thio treatment is essential.

Relaxers such as sodium bromide or calcium hydroxide cannot be used if thio products exist on the hair; they are similar to sodium hydroxide products, even though some are marketed as "no-lye" products. Think of the statement "no-lye" as a marketing tool, not as an absolute truth.

Calcium hydroxide relaxers must be mixed with an activator prior to their use. (The strength of the product can be adjusted by using more or less activator.) A calcium hydroxide relaxer is an option for the client who is allergic to sodium hydroxide.

Acid relaxers act like acid permanent waves, working with bisulfites rather than thioglycolate acid. These relaxers are designed to work mildly, and some can be used as a prewrap preparation for performing a curly perm on extremely curly hair. They are NOT compatible with sodium hydroxide or lye-based relaxers. In addition, potassium hydroxide relaxers are being developed—in part for clients who have sensitive scalps or allergies to other hydroxide-family products. They were initially extremely difficult to stabilize, although some are now being tried out.

With any relaxing or straightening product, read the manufacturer's directions carefully; different products vary widely. Also, use the neutralizing shampoo (also called a stabilizer or fixative) recommended by the manufacturer for optimum results. The neutralizer stops the action of any chemical relaxer that may remain on the hair after rinsing. The neutralizer for a thio-based relaxer reforms the cross-bonds in their new position and "rehardens" the hair. With lye-based products, think of the concept of neutralizing as less literal; the shampoos simply remove the relaxer from the hair.

PRE AND POST MUSTS

Prior to relaxing, the client's hairline must be protected with a petroleum base cream. This cream (or cream conditioner) can also be used during a relaxer touch-up to protect the previously relaxed hair and prevent overlapping of the product. In some instances, you may want to base the scalp to protect it from the product, particularly if the scalp is somewhat sensitive. If you opt to base the scalp, take straight partings and be careful not to get the base cream on the hair. Many of today's hydroxide-based relaxing products are "no-base" formulas, meaning that they have a built-in base that protects the scalp.

Relaxers are most frequently applied to the hair with the back of a comb or a brush; glove-covered hands can also be used, although this technique does not allow precise control of the product. Apply the product to the most resistant area first and the least resistant area last.

After relaxing, the hair must be rinsed thoroughly so that all the relaxer residue is rinsed out of the hair before the shampoo or neutralizer is applied. To rinse thoroughly, use warm water (never hot) and remove all the relaxer, paying particular attention to the hairline and the neck, where it rests against the sink. Wipe the rim of the sink periodically to make certain you are not repositioning the client's neckline onto a sink rim that has relaxing product on it. Then shampoo with the neutralizing or manufacturer-prescribed shampoo, turning the client's head to the left and right and washing the hairline and nape thoroughly. Rinse and shampoo a second time; then proceed with conditioning and styling.

RELAXING PROS AND CONS

Relaxers can be used to straighten the hair or to reduce the natural curl by a predetermined percentage. Hair should never be relaxed 100 percent so that it is "bone straight," or it will lack body and become susceptible to chemical damage, dryness and breakage. The largest percentage any curl configuration should ever be reduced by is about 95 percent.

Hair can also be texturized, which is sometimes referred to as partial relaxing or a curl-reduction service. With careful observation, you can stop the action of the relaxer when the curl pattern has been reduced anywhere from 10 to 60 percent. (More than 60 percent is edging toward straightening, not texturizing.) This allows you to reduce the curl, leaving the hair wavy, slightly curly or moderately curly. Texturizing results in a more manageable curl pattern that can be styled without the use of hot rollers, blow dryers or a curling iron.

Many clients can benefit from relaxing and texturizing services. Any time a client has extreme curl that he or she finds unmanageable, texturizing or relaxing may be an option. If the client lives in a humid climate, chemically relaxed styles are easy to control because the humidity won't cause curl to revert, like it does when hair is pressed or temporarily straightened. Relaxed styles are also ideal for the active client who does not want to spend lots of time on daily styling.

Texturizing reduces the curl pattern by a predetermined percentage and allows clients who have extremely curly hair to have softer curl or waves. If you texturize using a thio product, the client can opt for a perm any time after the service.

Relaxing and texturizing services are not an option for the client who has an abraded scalp, severely damaged hair, bleached hair, hair with metallic dye on it or evidence of hair breakage and poor elasticity. Additionally, some clients eschew chemical services completely and prefer styles that utilize the hair's natural texture.

Both the client's desires and the hair and scalp analysis lead to the decision to use hair straighteners or not. The analysis is also the basis of your choice of products and product strengths. Porosity and elasticity are particularly important to observe when straightening hair. In general, the more porous the hair, the faster it will relax; the more resistant the hair, the longer it will take to relax. If elasticity is poor or porosity is extreme, the hair should not be relaxed. If you have any questions about the role of the analysis in making a relaxing-service decision, refer back to Chapter 4 and review the steps of the hair analysis.

PRODUCT STRENGTHS

The hair analysis and strand test will help you select the appropriate product strength. The curl pattern and the desired end result (along with the product's strength) will determine the timing of the service. Keep the following pointers in mind when making product selection and timing decisions:

◆ If hair is fine or tinted, use a mild strength product and always perform a strand test.

◆ Most medium-textured, curly hair that is in good condition will relax with a medium-strength product.

◆ If hair is very coarse and resistant, use a strong, or super-strength, product. Avoid this when possible by performing a strand test with a medium-strength product.

◆ In general, very tight curl is more porous and takes about thirteen to fifteen minutes to relax; coarse, resistant hair takes about eighteen to twenty minutes to relax.

◆ Extremely curly hair is frequently somewhat porous; curl that has an elongated curl or wave pattern is often more resistant. However, make no assumptions; perform a porosity test.

◆ Always read manufacturer's directions when choosing a relaxer strength and judging timing. Brands vary widely when it comes to recommended processing time and the hair type for which various strengths are recommended.

◆ Keep an eye on the hair at all times. When relaxing for a very straight effect, lift the strand to see if it buckles away the scalp, indicating hair is not 90 to 95 percent straightened. When texturizing, check to see whether or not the desired curl pattern has been achieved. Hair will often process at a faster or slower rate than the product manufacturer's guidelines indicate. Continually read the hair; never walk away and return to check the hair only after the manufacturer's recommended time has expired.

◆ If you mix the relaxer with oil, you can slow the relaxing process. Some stylists do this with mild relaxers to use them during texturizing services. Others add oil because they need more time to apply and smooth the product. (Recommended processing times include application and smoothing.) If you wish to try adding oil, add a small amount to the product that you'll be using immediately and mix thoroughly.

◆ Spot relaxing can be performed when the hairline is unruly or overly curly. Apply the product (carefully!) to the hairline only and you'll soften the edges, giving the hairline a softer look. Do not do this on a fragile hairline or if you see evidence of breakage.

◆ Do not comb through the hair if you wish to relax it to the maximum degree; simply smooth it. Do comb through the hair using a wide-toothed comb when texturizing. You'll want to observe the hair continuously to determine when it reaches the desired wave pattern.

PRECAUTIONS

Jon Rogers, of The Place for Hair and Face in Los Angeles, California, provides these additional tips for safe relaxing:

◆ Even if you are familiar with the client and his or her hair, perform a hair and scalp analysis prior to every chemical service.

◆ Avoid shampooing prior to relaxing. Shampooing makes the scalp especially sensitive to relaxing products.

◆ Always perform a stand test prior to relaxing. Apply the product to a few strands at the nape, and leave it on for at least fifteen minutes but no longer than twenty. Rinse, shampoo and test the strands to determine the hair's elasticity. If good elasticity exists, you can proceed with the service.

◆ Prior to texturizing, check the hair for inconsistent curl patterns. Determine where the tightest curl exists and begin the product application at that area.

◆ Always wear gloves when applying relaxers or straightening products.

◆ Always apply a protective cream to the hairline prior to using hair straighteners.

◆ Frequently take a test curl to determine the action of the product, regardless of manufacturer-stated processing times.

◆ Always rinse thoroughly before neutralizing. Sodium relaxer has an oil base that reacts with the shampoo and penetrates the hair. If you shampoo prematurely, the oil will become extremely difficult to remove. If this occurs, blow dry the hair, apply talcum powder, comb it through and shampoo again.

◆ Cellophanes and jazzing hair colors can be used immediately after relaxing. They do not contain any peroxide or use activators that do. The freshly relaxed hair is porous, so it will rapidly absorb the color.

◆ If the client wants relaxer and haircolor, perform the relaxing service first. Perform the color service a week later; to stay on the safe side, limit the service to a single-step process that uses semi- or demi-permanent products.

◆ Never bleach hair that has been relaxed.

◆ In the case of a chemical burn, apply ice immediately. If a blister rises, send the client to a dermatologist.

VIRGIN RELAXER SERVICE

During a virgin relaxing service, the hair is straightened using the relaxing product and minimal mechanical action. It is not necessary to use the teeth of the comb; mechanical action should be limited to smoothing with the glove-covered fingers or pressing with the back of the comb.

Always analyze the hair and pre-test a few strands at the nape of the neck prior to performing a relaxing service. Make certain the hair is completely dry prior to relaxing, and place the client under a cool dryer for five to ten minutes if there is any doubt. Then use this simple technique from Jon Rogers at the Place for Hair and Face in Los Angeles:

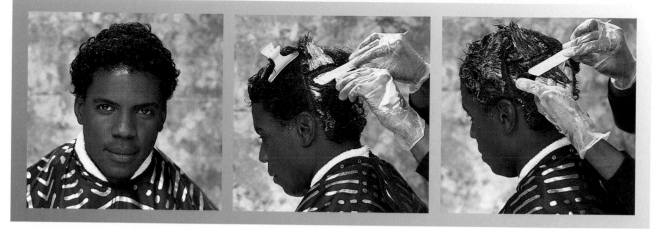

FIGURE 10.1
Apply protective cream around the hairline.

FIGURE 10.2
Using a brush or the back of a comb, apply the relaxer.

FIGURE 10.3
Press the strand firmly between the comb and your gloved hand.

1. First apply protective cream around the hairline, from back to front and around the ears. (Fig. 10.1) Cover the parts of the ears that could be exposed to the relaxer. If the client has single-process haircolor, use a mild product; if the curl pattern is extreme and the hair somewhat porous, use a medium-strength product; if the hair is wavy or resistant, use a super-strength product. If the client may want a curl later or if you want a milder product that's less irritating to the scalp, use a thio-based relaxer.

2. Section the hair into four parts. Begin applying the relaxer at the most resistant area, using the same application procedure as you would for a first-time tint service. Beginning at the back crown, apply the relaxer to the hair, section by section. Use a brush or the back of the comb and apply the product one-quarter inch from the scalp to the ends. (Fig. 10.2)

3. Work from the crown to the nape, then move in a clockwise direction to the next section.

4. When the back is completed, apply the product to the front, working from the crown to the temples on both sides.

5. Once the application is complete, begin to speed straightening of the hair, using a mechanical, smoothing action. Move back to your starting point at the crown and, working from crown to nape, press the strand firmly between the back of the rattail comb and your gloved hand. (Fig. 10.3) Move the comb downward from the scalp to the ends of the strand, pressing it against the hand that holds the section of hair. Do not use the teeth of the comb.

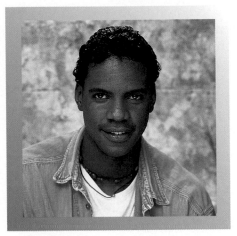

FIGURE 10.4
Finished style, "virgin relaxer service."

6. Repeat the procedure throughout the back and in the front, from crown to temple. Follow the same pattern that you used to apply the product, pressing the hair against your hand, section by section.

7. When the smoothing procedure is completed, check the first section to which you applied the product to see if the desired degree of relaxing has been achieved. Check your manufacturer's directions for processing time, but check the hair periodically as well, particularly if it is porous. For total straightening (as opposed to texturizing) relax the hair by about 90 percent. The strand should not buckle against the scalp when lifted; it should lie smoothly, but not be 100 percent straight.

8. When processing is complete, rinse the relaxing product out thoroughly and shampoo twice with the prescribed neutralizing shampoo.

HAIR TEXTURIZING AND SHAPING

The procedure for texturizing is similar to that for relaxing, only when texturizing the hair, do gently comb through it, using a large-toothed comb. This allows you to observe the curl pattern as it releases and halt processing when the desired degree of curl reduction is achieved.

The following technique, from Jon Rogers at the Place for Hair and Face in Los Angeles, uses sodium hydroxide; therefore the hair should not have been shampooed for twenty-four hours prior to the service. If the hair has semi-permanent color, always use a mild-strength relaxer; do not texturize hair that has been bleached or colored using a double process.

First, make certain the hair and scalp are completely dry. If there is any question about dampness, place the client under a cool dryer for five to ten minutes prior to texturizing. In this instance, the pattern of extremely curly hair will be reduced by 50 percent to leave softer curl with strong wave. The short style is then reshaped into a style that takes advantage of the softened wave.

1. The natural curl pattern is extremely curly and the hair is longer at the top and shorter at the back and sides. To begin, apply a protective cream around the hairline from nape to front. Then cover the ears with the cream anywhere they might touch the relaxing product.

2. Beginning at the crown, apply the product to the hair, section by section. If the hair is extremely dense, take smaller sections. Start one-quarter inch from the scalp and apply the product along the section, using the back of a large-toothed comb. Work from the crown to the nape; then move in a clockwise direction to the next section. Apply the relaxer on the surface and underside of the strand, using the comb to evenly distribute the product.

3. When the back is completed, apply the product from the crown to the temple, working all the way to the front hairline. Once all the hair has been covered with the product, check for even distribution, lifting the hair with your glove-covered hands. Work the product into any areas that you missed. Then wait two to three minutes for the hair to soften before you attempt combing through the hair.

4. Now begin to mechanically relax the hair to the desired curl pattern by gently combing the hair from scalp to ends. Start combing where hair is least resistant; allow the product to continue softening the most resistant hair while you do this. Avoid excess tension, and gently comb from front to back, as far as the hair will allow you to go without using force. Then continue by combing the resistant area. When you have combed through the hair, lift it up, allowing it to buckle down slightly, and observe the curl pattern. (Use the back of the comb to smooth excess relaxing product out of the way, so that you can closely observe the curl pattern.)

5. Once the desired curl pattern is achieved, wait about thirty more seconds to allow the dried hair to contract a bit. Then rinse thoroughly and neutralize, using a prescribed neutralizing shampoo. Next shampoo a second time. Towel dry the hair and begin reshaping, cutting the nape close. Work up the back of the head to the center back.

6. Create a slight increase above the center back by angling your fingers. The top will be left longer. Then square off the back and lift all the lower lengths with the comb to make certain that they are even.

7. Next taper the hair around the ears, angling the shears to create a sharp sideburn line. Cut the first inch or so close to the head, matching the back length.

8. An inch-and-a-half to two inches above the top of the ear, begin angling your fingers to create a length increase. Use this line as a guide to complete the uniformly layered, longer top.

9. Complete both sides in the same manner. In this case, the hair will be worn asymmetrically, so the weight line at the heavier side is sharply defined.

10. The hair can now be blown dry, using a large-diameter round brush, and iron curled for soft texture. Other variations include gelling the completed cut and allowing it to dry naturally or setting the longer top on small-sized Velcro rollers.

RELAXER TOUCH-UP

Six to eight weeks after a relaxing service, depending on the hair's rate of growth, the hair will need a relaxer touch-up at the regrowth area. This should be done when the hair has grown out approximately three-quarters of an inch to one inch. Do not attempt a touch-up service if there is not sufficient regrowth present or if there is evidence of hair breakage or scalp problems.

Jon Rogers, of the Place for Hair and Face in Los Angeles, recommends approaching the relaxer touch-up service the same way as you would a tint touch-up service. Here is his simple technique:

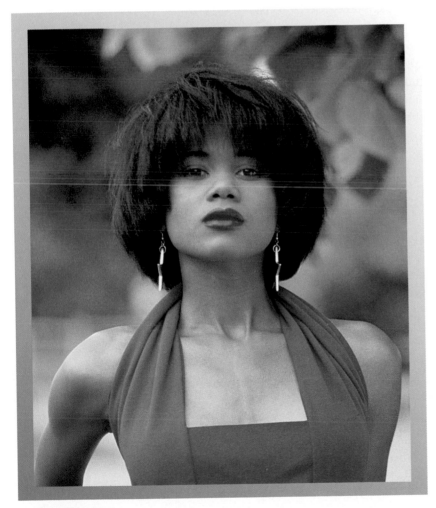

FIGURE 10.5
Relaxed hair with texturized ends. Image: Aveda.

1. Examine the hair and scalp before proceeding with the service. If there are no contraindications, apply protective cream around the hairline from back to front. Also, apply the cream to the top, back and perimeter of the ears.

2. Section the hair into four parts and begin applying the relaxer at the crown, using the back of a rattail comb to smooth on the product.

3. Begin applying the product as close to the scalp as possible, but do not touch the scalp with the product.

4. Work down to the nape, taking care not to overlap the relaxer onto the previously relaxed hair. Confine the product to the new growth only.

5. Work from the crown to the nape, taking vertical partings throughout the back and applying the product. Smooth it onto all the regrowth with the back of the comb.

6. When the back is completed, move to the crown, take a horizontal parting and apply the relaxer to the regrowth only.

7. Continue taking horizontal sections and applying the relaxer from the temple, across the top of the head to the crown and down to the opposite temple.

8. Work toward the front hairline, continuing to take partings from the temple to the crown. Complete the application by applying the relaxer to the front hairline.

9. Check the regrowth to make certain the relaxer is smoothed on evenly and resmooth sections as needed.

10. Press the hairline firmly with the comb to ensure even processing, but do not comb through the hair. Process until the hair has relaxed the desired amount, then rinse thoroughly with warm water. Make certain all the relaxer residue is removed, then shampoo twice and condition.

A WORD ABOUT CURL RESTRUCTURING

Note:

Many conditioners on the market today are referred to as hair restructors or "reconstructors" and are not to be confused with a curl restructuring service; always make certain you and your client are discussing the same thing. If the client wants to go from a curly perm to straight hair, explain the difficulties and the options.

Some manufacturers claim that their products permit the client to go from a curly perm back to straightened hair or vice versa. If a client's hair has been straightened or texturized using a thio-based product, the client does have the option of getting a perm later. However, it is never recommended that you try to take a client from a perm back to straight hair. Severe hair breakage is the most likely result of such an attempt.

If your client wants to return to straightened hair, the permed hair must be grown out. Then hair can be cut short, as guided by the regrowth, and the regrowth can be straightened or relaxed. Until sufficient regrowth is achieved, thermal pressing or heat styling is the safest option for creating a straight style.

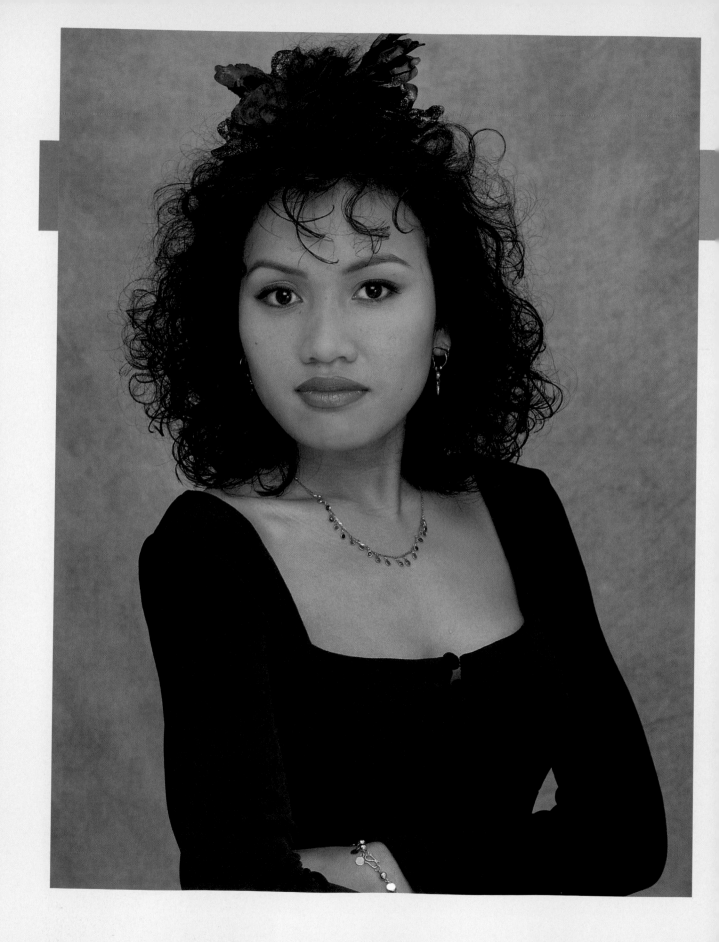

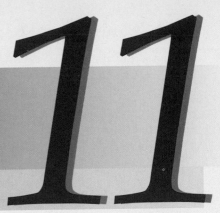
One- and Two-Step Perms and Advanced Perming Techniques

As an advanced stylist, you should already be familiar with the theories and principles of perming. In general, with the one-step perm, acid waves are best for long hair, hair that has been previously permed or porous hair. Alkaline perms require no heat and process quickly; therefore, they are best for normal to resistant hair.

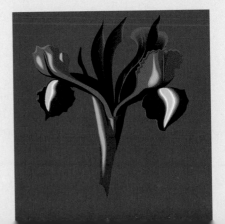

Exothermic perms, which are self-heating and self-timing, take a longer time to process but avoid over-processing. Special perms exist for color-treated and bleached hair; if you used higher than 20 volume developer, opt for the bleached-hair formulation.

When it comes to perming today, more perming products and tools than ever can be used to achieve a wide variety of curl patterns on different hair types.

ONE-STEP PERMING OF COARSE OR FINE HAIR

Two types of hair will require special consideration when you perform a one-step perm. If the hair is coarse and resistant, select a perm that achieves the desired results in the shortest period of time to avoid excess chemical stress and over-processing. Over-processing is the most common error stylists make when perming coarse, resistant hair.

When used correctly, an **alkaline perm**, which is stronger, faster acting and does not require heat, is usually the best choice. Additionally, according to educator James Christopher Chan, of the The Hair Resort in Las Vegas, Nevada, classic Asian hair should not be permed on small rods. When the rods are smaller, the hair's bonds have farther to shift, and the result could be a frizzy looking perm. Instead, opt for larger rods, which will give you smoother results.

When perming fine, straight hair, many stylists erroneously assume it will take a long time to perm. Again the tendency is toward over-processing. One problem is that fine, slightly wavy hair looks straight to the eye when it is dried naturally, but the bonds actually have a characteristic of being wavy and the hair will curl quickly. To test the hair, shampoo it, then take a cluster of ends, pull on them and release them. If they snap back and stand up straight, the bonds are aligned in such a way that the hair is truly straight, and it will be harder to perm. If they do not stand up straight, the hair may be easier to perm.

PERMING DOUBLE-PROCESSED HAIR

Hair that has been colored using a double process can be permed, using a single-step perming process. Generally, you should perm prior to coloring because perming solution will lighten haircolor.

Specific perms on the market today are especially formulated for use with double-processed hair. Perform a complete hair and scalp analysis first to determine whether there are contraindications, such as excess porosity, breakage or scalp sensitivity. Prior to the perm, during the procedure and after toning, hair should be reconditioned. Further precautions include:

◆ Use larger-diameter rods, which place less chemical stress on hair because bonds do not have to shift as far.
◆ Wrap the hair with multiple end-papers. Use a "cushion wrapping" technique, in which end papers are placed all along the strand so that hair never rests directly on other hair. This diminishes the trauma that can occur when perm solution penetrates quickly.
◆ Use buffered perm solutions and remoisturizers. Avoid hydrolyzed animal protein conditioners, which can leech out moisture.
◆ If you use a cold (alkaline) wave, dilute the solution by 50 percent with distilled water, then add buffers, such as a remoisturizer. Wrap with minimal or no tension. Using a low-pH acid wave may give more satisfactory results.
◆ Always use picks to lift the bands of the rods off of the hair. Continuously observe the curl and take test curls frequently. Double-processed hair can actually take a curl in as little as sixty seconds.

TWO-STEP PERMING

The two-step perm is a process by which very curly hair is transformed into larger, softer curl. In the one-step perm, you begin with straight hair; in the two-step perm, you begin with very curly hair; therefore, you must straighten it first and then create a new curl configuration in a second step. The new curl will be determined by the size of the rod and the wrapping technique, just as it is with the one-step perm.

As noted in Chapter 10, the products used must be compatible. In the two-step perm, hair can only be straightened with a thio-based product since permanent-waving solution contains thioglycolic acid.

The perming solution used in the two-step perm is almost identical to the perming solution used in the single-step perm; the primary difference is that the two-step perm solution tends to be stronger.

The steps are very simple: relax the hair with a thio product, rinse thoroughly, apply a conditioner or a perming solution, wrap the hair on rods, process and neutralize. As with the one-step perm, you can either wrap the hair with water and apply the perming solution after wrapping, or wrap the hair with the solution. Curly hair that has been straightened with a thio-based product can also be molded into a new shape, as opposed to being wrapped on rods.

Wrapping the hair is sometimes called *rodding* the hair in the African-American community; the two-step perm itself is referred to as a *cold-wave*, a *body perm*, or, simply, a *curl*. It is also frequently called by the name of the product itself, for example, a *Jheri curl*. The thio-based straightening product or relaxer is sometimes called a *reducing cream* or a *curl rearranger*. The perm solution itself is most often called a *curl booster*.

As mentioned, some stylists wrap the hair with the booster or perm solution, which helps soften the hair so it can be wrapped more easily with the correct amount of tension. This is particularly helpful if the hair is fine; the technique is also used in the one-step perm. If you wrap the hair with a perming solution, dilute the solution and apply it to the hair section-by-section. Process according to directions, rinse thoroughly, allow the client to sit in the open air for twenty to thirty minutes, then chemically neutralize.

For hair of average texture, the hair is usually wrapped with water prior to applying the perm solution or booster, then each rod is saturated with the perming solution. Wrapping with water or solution is often a personal choice; let experience be your guide.

The perming solution or booster, when used in the two-step process, is often called "curl insurance" because it leaves nothing to chance. The hair can be curled after it is straightened without using the booster. For example, curly hair can be straightened, then oxidized on the rods, and it will take on the new curl formation without the use of a perming solution or booster. (In this instance, wrap the hair quickly, before it begins to oxidize. If it takes you longer than twenty to twenty-five minutes to wrap all the hair, use a perm solution or booster.) Perming solution should always be used when hair is resistant.

If you wrap the hair with conditioner and do not use the solution as your "curl insurance," comb the conditioner through the hair completely, wrap the hair on rods and cover the client's head with a plastic cap. Place him or her under the dryer for fifteen minutes to speed penetration of the conditioner, then allow the hair to air oxidize for an additional fifteen minutes. When the desired curl pattern has been achieved, rinse the hair and chemically neutralize it to lock the new curl in place and return the hair to its natural pH.

A few salons still use air oxidation or air drying to neutralize the curl, instead of using a chemical neutralizer. When air neutralizing, the rods must be left in the hair for twenty-four hours. While this can be done with either the one- or two-step perm, and can be gentler on hair, the technique is rarely employed since it is not practical for the client.

These variations—allowing the hair to air neutralize and wrapping with conditioner instead of a curl booster—are performed to avoid extra chemical exposure and to minimize drying from the thio-based perm solution. Thio products tend to be very drying on hair—particularly when it has been treated twice by relaxing and then perming.

ONE- AND TWO-STEP PERMING BY HAIR TYPE

Any type of hair can be permed to create either a softer or a tighter-than-natural curl. Use the following hair-type chart as a general guide to using a one or two-step perm.

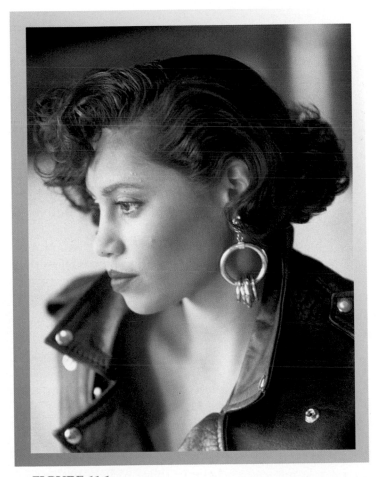

FIGURE 11.1
Creating a soft curl. Hair: Fran Cotter for John Paul Mitchell Systems; Photo: Jack Cutler.

RESISTANT, CURLY HAIR

1. Reduce curl with a thio-based straightener.
2. Wrap the hair on rods with a curl booster. (Variation for adding new curl.)
3. Process.
4. Rinse, blot and neutralize.

WAVY, MODERATELY RESISTANT HAIR

1. Reduce curl with a thio-based straightener.
2. Wrap the hair on rods.
3. Air oxidize.
4. Rinse, blot and neutralize.

VERY FINE, THIN, STRAIGHT HAIR

1. Wrap the hair with an acid or cold-wave solution, using minimal tension.
2. Rinse, blot and neutralize.

ROD SIZES AND POSITIONING

Whether you are performing a one- or a two-step perm, the curl you create will be determined by the size of the rod and the wrapping technique that you use. In general, the smaller the rod, the more curl you'll achieve; the larger the rod, the more wave or body you will achieve—or the less curl you'll get. Therefore, pink, gray and white rods create curl; purple rods create body.

The rods' position within the base affects results, just as it does with a roller set. Refer to the section in Chapter 8 entitled "Base Control" to refresh your memory as to the relationship between a tool and base on which it rests. In general, on-base positioning creates volume; off-base positioning produces less volume and a weaker curl. Over-direction creates maximum volume, while under-direction results in less volume.

Mix up tool sizes and wrapping techniques, and you can create a variety of curl patterns within a single hair design.

ADVANCED WRAPPING TECHNIQUES

Perm wrapping techniques can be extremely creative. While conventional perm wrapping is performed from ends to scalp, there are many other ways to create customized curl. Hair can be spiralled around a roller to create ringlets. If you wrap only the hair near the scalp, you get a "root" perm or lift at the scalp. With this technique, you can either leave the ends free or wrap them on a different-sized rod for a design wrap.

What follows are just a few advanced perm-wrapping techniques that are used to create a specific curl configuration, contrast within a single design, curl expansion or curl compression. When you use these wrapping techniques, always plan the complete hair design in advance and design the perm wrap to work in conjunction with the final hair cut.

BRICKLAYING

Bricklaying is one of the most common wraps that eliminates part lines and separation between curls. (Using zig-zag partings also eliminates the "separated-curl" effect that is particularly common with fine hair.)

To bricklay rods, wrap the front hairline first, directing the hair off the face. Move back one row and center these rods in the spaces

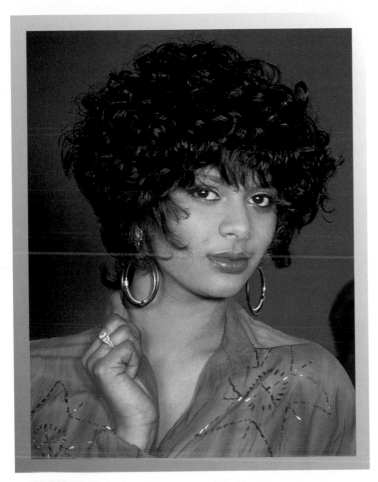

FIGURE 11.2
Creating customized curl. Hair: Fran Cotter for John Paul Mitchell Systems; Photo: Jack Cutler.

between the rods at the hairline. They should look the same way bricks do when they are laid, meaning that no rod is positioned directly behind the other. Continue wrapping hair in this manner, each time positioning the rod so that only half of it is behind the rod in front of it.

You can create a bricklay pattern anywhere on the head; for example, you can use it at the top of the occipital only, where hair often separates or "splits." Regardless of where you begin wrapping the hair, you can bricklay the rods behind your first row. The example used, in which wrapping begins at the front hairline, is for a style in which the hair moves away from the face.

PIGGYBACK WRAPPING

The piggyback wrap uses two or more rods for each section of hair. It requires hair that is at least six inches long and can be performed to create stronger end curl or scalp wave. It also helps the lotion penetrate coarse, resistant hair more easily. It is an excellent technique for hair that is very dense, which would otherwise require that you wrap very small sections.

To create it, begin with a usual-sized parting of about a half-inch. Wrap the hair from the center of the strand to the scalp, using one rod. Then take a second, smaller rod and wrap the hair from the ends down to the first rod. Insert a toothpick between the bands of both rods to hold them together and to keep the bands off of the hair.

For even curl, use rods that are all the same size. For end curl, use a larger rod closest to the scalp and a smaller one at the ends. For a stronger wave at the scalp and looser end curl, use a medium-sized rod from center strand to the scalp and a larger-sized one from the center of the strand to the ends.

ALTERNATING WRAPS

For jumbled-up curl, wrap hair in the conventional fashion, from ends to scalp, but alternate the direction of every other rod. For example, begin at the hairline, wrapping the rod away from the face. Then, wrap the next rod toward the face. Continue this alternating pattern throughout the entire head. This technique can be used on hair that is anywhere from two to six inches long. The shorter the hair, the more evident the tousled curls will be.

STACK WRAPPING

Stack wrapping works best for mid-length hair that contains no more than minimal layering at the front. It creates varying amounts of end curl because the rods "stack" up and out from the nape at an angle. They are held in place and supported by long sticks, such as chopsticks or long coffee stirrers. As you move up the head from the nape, less and less of each strand is wrapped, because it travels from the top, across the curve of the head, and then downward to reach the stacked rods.

First, wrap horizontal sections at the nape, beginning at the hairline. Wrap the rods on-base, from the ends up to the scalp. After three or four rods have been wrapped, determine the angle of the stack by taking a strand of hair at the crown. Hold it straight out and back, then determine how far from the ends the rod will be wrapped on this strand. Base your decision on the amount of end curl desired and the final form. (Hair at the scalp will not be wrapped.)

Once you determine where along this strand you will position the rod, bring the strand down while still holding it out from the head. Take the sticks that the rods will rest against and position them under the elastic bands of the previously wrapped rods. They should move upward and out at an angle. Now bring the strand from the crown down and allow it to meet the supporting sticks at the point where the partially wrapped roller will sit. If the top strand will be wrapped to within a few inches from the scalp, you will have to push the sticks toward the head to create a steeper angle. If only a few inches of the strand at the crown will be wrapped, position the sticks so they move farther away from the head to meet the crown strand at the point at which you'll stop wrapping the roller. In either case, you are establishing the angle of the stack that will serve as your wrapping guide. Keep this angle in mind, should you move the sticks out of place.

To complete wrapping, work up the head, under-directing each rod so it just reaches the sticks that hold all the rods. Begin at the ends, hold the hair out and wrap the rod up to where the sticks, or "stabilizers," are placed. Slide the rod's bands over the sticks. When you reach the top, each rod will rest on the one below it and will be positioned farther out from the head. Repeat the procedure all around the head.

You can reverse the procedure so the rods stack straight outward from the bottom to achieve an entirely different effect.

BODY WRAPS FOR SHORT HAIR

To create a body wave on short hair, use large-sized rods and wrap them in the direction that you want the hair to move. (Again, this should be pre-planned with the final cut in mind.) Often, when you reach the short nape hair, it will not wrap more than half a revolution or so around the rod. While many stylists leave this hair unpermed or wrap it on smaller rods, a better solution may be to wrap the hair into large pin curls. Then the longer hair will move into the shorter lengths in a more fluid fashion, and you will not have excess curl at the nape or perimeter. The entire head can also be permed in large pin curls, for yet another curl configuration. Pin curls, like rollers and perm rods, sit on a base and can be designed for a variety of looks.

PERMING PRECAUTIONS

With a thorough understanding of perming techniques, perming products and the hair type with which you are working, you can create a variety of curl types. Always perform a hair analysis first and base your decisions on the hair's condition and the client's desires.

If a two-step perm is to be performed, be sure that the client understands that the hair cannot be chemically straightened after the perm. The hair must be grown out. Hair that has been permed using the two-step process cannot be blow dried, thermally set or pressed on a regular basis without significantly weakening the newly created curl pattern. If the consultation reveals that versatility is the client's true aim, suggest the hair be relaxed and thermally or mechanically styled to achieve a variety of looks.

Since thio-based products tend to be drying to the hair, whenever perming, recommend that the client regularly condition and remoisturize the hair. This is particularly important if the hair has been permed using a two-step process. When the hair has been straightened and then curled, overuse of some protein products will cause the hair to appear to revert to its natural state.

ADVANCED PERMING TECHNIQUES

VIRGIN TWO-STEP PERM FOR CURLY HAIR

When hair is extremely curly, a perm gives the hair more body, creates controlled curl and a softer feel, adds manageability and allows the client to enjoy relatively maintenance-free styling. Prior to the service, the hair should be in good condition, contain no sodium hydroxide product, and be free of metallic dyes, bleach and henna compounds. If the hair has any color on it at all, perform a test curl prior to the service.

The following technique, from Jon Rogers of The Place for Hair and Face in Los Angeles, is for virgin hair that has not been previously exposed to relaxer, permanent-wave products or haircolor. It presents the ideal situation, exemplifying the proper steps and procedures. If the client has had any previous chemical services, adjust this procedure accordingly, perform a test curl and refuse the service if you find contraindications.

1. Shampoo the hair lightly using a pH-balanced shampoo. Rinse, towel dry and apply a protective cream around the entire perimeter of the hairline. Remove tangles with a large-toothed comb, then section the hair into four or five subsections.

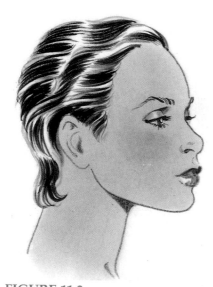

FIGURE 11.3
The hair is completely covered with the straightener. Illustrations: Milady's Standard Textbook of Cosmetology.

2. Put on protective gloves and begin applying the thio-based straightening product at the nape or the most resistant area. Take a half-inch parting and apply the product from near the scalp to the ends, using the back of a rattail comb to smooth on the product. Do not comb through the strand or press the comb hard against it.

3. Work from the nape to the crown, or crown to nape, depending on which area is most resistant. Then move to the front and apply the product from the temples to the front hairline.

4. When all the hair has been completely covered with the straightener, cover the hairline with a strip of protective cotton and place a plastic bag over the client's head. (Fig. 11.3) (Do not use a bag that has contains any elastic, such as a shower cap; the elastic can cause painful burns at the hairline.) Then place the client under a dryer to soften the virgin hair. Depending on how tight the original curl pattern is, the client should remain under the dryer from five to ten minutes. (If the hair is not virgin, do not place the client under the dryer.)

5. Next remove the client from under the dryer and check the hair for softness. Then continue with the straightening process. Begin at your original starting point and use a wide-toothed comb to gently comb through each section. Taking care not to touch the scalp with the teeth of the comb, pull the comb through the section of hair from close to the scalp to the

ends. Continue combing and mechanically straightening from scalp to ends, as you retrace your original application pattern.

6. When the hair is supple and flexible, rinse the hair thoroughly to remove all traces of the thio straightener. If you believe that any chemical persists in the hair, lightly shampoo. (Follow the manufacturer's directions; some vary regarding this step.)

7. Next, apply a pre-wrap solution and begin wrapping the hair on the rods you have pre-selected, based on the desired curl pattern. Wrap each section tightly and smoothly around the rod; the way it lies is the way it will look when you remove the rods.

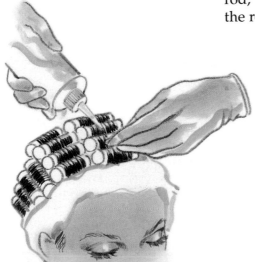

FIGURE 11.4
Carefully apply the waving solution to each rod.

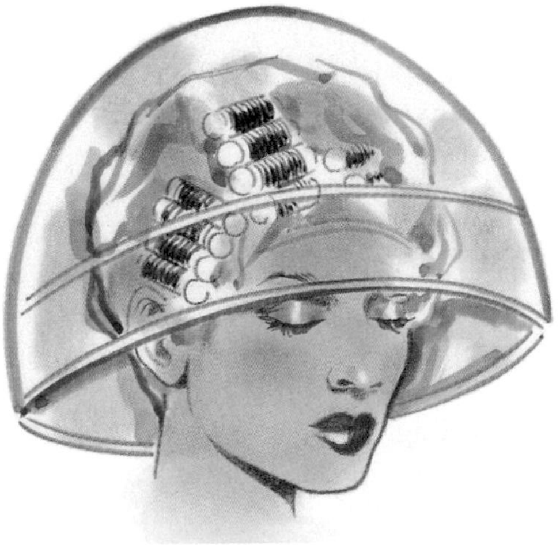

8. Generously reapply the protective creme around the hairline and place a strip of cotton completely around the hairline from front to back. Then mix the waving solution and carefully apply it to each rod, saturating both the top and underside of each rod. (Fig. 11.4) Avoid applying the product to the scalp. (If the manufacturer's directions have not called for the thio straightener to be rinsed out, at this point spray each rod with liquid waving lotion to re-activate the thio product.)

9. After applying the perming solution, remove the wet cotton. The chemical-soaked cotton could burn the client's skin if left in place. Replace the cotton with a fresh, dry strip and place a plastic bag over the client's head. Then place the client under a preheated dryer for fifteen to twenty-five minutes, as specified by the manufacturer. (Fig. 11.5) (If hair is not virgin or is porous, check the hair prior to the recommended timing.)

10. Check the curl pattern by gently unwinding the rod one-and-a-half revolutions, without pulling on the hair. (Fig. 11.6) Re-test the curl regularly; if it has not achieved the desired pattern at the end of the manufacturer-specified time, reapply the perming solution, change the protective cotton strip, and place the client back under the dryer. (Test the curl very frequently if you have reapplied the solution.)

11. When the desired curl pattern has been achieved, rinse the hair thoroughly, taking

FIGURE 11.5
Cover the hair with a plastic bag, and place the client under the dryer.

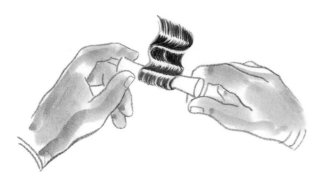

FIGURE 11.6
Check the curl pattern.

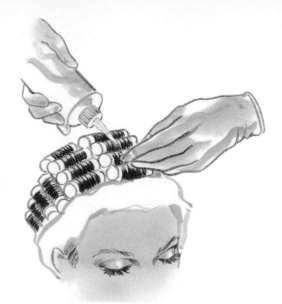

FIGURE 11.7
After rinsing, apply the neutralizer.

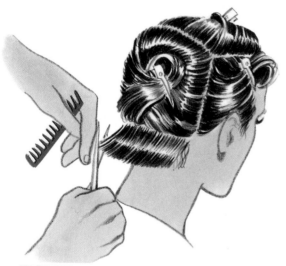

FIGURE 11.8
Trim and shape the hair.

care not to disturb the rods, towel blot each rod, apply the neutralizer and process according to the manufacturer's directions. (Fig. 11.7) Usually neutralizing takes five to ten minutes. (Some manufacturers recommend spritzing on liquid conditioner prior to neutralizing; read instructions carefully.)

12. After neutralizing, carefully remove the rods, or rinse and then remove the rods, based on the manufacturer's directions. Gently towel dry, then trim and shape the hair, and style as desired. (Fig. 11.8)

CURLY PERM TOUCH-UP

The curly perm touch-up is often called a recurl. To perform a recurl, follow the same procedure for the touch-up as you did for the initial application—with one exception. When you apply the thio-based straightener, apply it to the new growth only. Avoid overlapping the product onto the previously curled hair by taking extra care during the application and covering the previously curled hair with a protective cream or a thick conditioner. When you wrap the hair and apply the perm solution or curl booster, the previously permed hair remains protected by the cream conditioner. (Reapply after straightening if necessary.) You can also use a "root" perm technique, if the desired curl configuration permits.

Prior to each recurl service, trim the ends and perform a porosity test. Always use a product that is compatible with the original one used. Partial or complete air oxidation during the neutralizing phase protects the hair further.

THE STRAIGHT PERM

The straight perm technique uses an ammonium thioglycolate perm solution to straighten naturally curly hair. Because the solution is not as strong as a relaxing product, the service is potentially less damaging to hair, but it is limited to fine to medium-textured hair. Do not try this technique with extremely coarse or excessively curly hair.

It is not recommended that you try to straighten chemically curled hair primarily because sodium relaxers are incompatible with thio-based curling products. In addition, the excess chemical stress of trying to revert curl almost ensures hair breakage. However, Karen Lafferty, who is the regional training manager for Creative Hairdressers, Inc., Falls Church, Virginia, uses the straight perm technique to straighten permanently waved hair, when the hair's porosity and elasticity are good. Always perform tests for elasticity and porosity prior to using a straight perm technique.

The straight perm technique requires that the perming solution be applied to the hair against a hard surface. While many stylists use long plastic strips to create a straight perm, Lafferty uses the surface of the head in a technique similar to the one used to style "the wrap," which is described in Chapter 9. It's simple to perform and eliminates the need to purchase the long plastic strips.

1. To begin, examine the hair and perform elasticity and porosity tests. Then shampoo the hair with a clarifying shampoo to remove any product build-up.

2. Section off the front from the back with a parting that moves from ear-to-ear, across the top of the head. Then slice off a one-inch section at the nape.

3. Mix the perming solution with equal parts of a moisturizing conditioner. Using a tint brush, apply the mixture to the hair, beginning at the nape. Brush on the mixture, then comb through the hair with a wide-toothed comb to ensure even distribution.

4. Next move up the head and release another one-inch parting. Repeat the application procedure, combing through the hair gently. Continue to work up the back, then continue through the front, repeating the application and combing procedures.

5. When the mixture has been applied to all of the hair, begin wrapping the hair. Using a small-toothed comb or the end of a rattail comb, take a low side parting and wrap the section around the head, using moderate tension.

6. Continue slicing off sections and wrapping them back over the previously wrapped section until you have molded the hair all the way around the head. (Fig. 11.9)

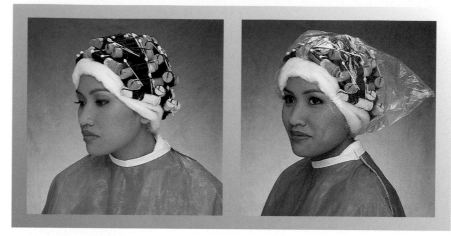

FIGURE 11.9
Continue the procedure until all the hair has been wrapped.

FIGURE 11.10
Cover the hair with a plastic cap and process.

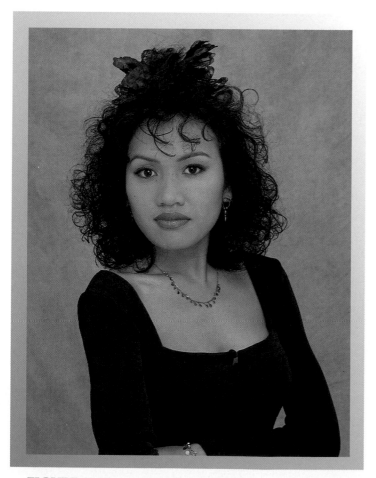

FIGURE 11.11
Finished style, "Straight perm." Photo: Sally Russ for SalonOvations' Beautiful Black Styles.

7. Cover the hair with a plastic cap and process, based on manufacturer's instructions and the desired degree of curl reduction. (Fig. 11.10)

8. When processing is complete, rinse the hair with tepid water for at least 5 minutes. Towel-blot the hair, taking care not to scrunch it.

9. Now, starting at the nape, apply the neutralizer to the hair section-by-section. Work from the nape, up the head, to the front hairline. Comb the neutralizer through the hair, using a wide-toothed comb; then rewrap the hair in the opposite direction it was previously wrapped.

10. Allow the neutralizer to remain in the hair for five minutes. Then rinse thoroughly and apply a deep-moisturizing treatment. After rinsing out the moisturizer, proceed with styling by sculpting the hair, air drying or blow drying.

TEXTURIZING PERMS

Coarse, resistant hair, whether curly or straight, can achieve natural-looking curl when permed using irregular-sized sections for the wrap. In the following technique, hair at the front fringe or bang area is left un-permed, for a textural mix. This approach also allows you to perm hair that has a fragile front hairline. Some sections at the center top are also left un-permed, allowing the un-permed bangs to better blend into the design. The back is wrapped tightly, using irregularly-shaped, smaller-than-normal partings.

If the hair is extremely curly, it should be straightened with a thio-based product prior to performing the perm. The wrapping technique presented here is ideal for coarse hair that is cut short or contains light layering. The product used is an alkaline perm that is especially formulated for resistant, coarse or hard-to-curl hair.

The perming technique was created by Mary Light for Interzone and Zotos Ultra Bond, Ultra Cool Permanent Wave. It requires the use of picks or rod "stabilizers" to keep the elastic bands off of the hair and secure the rods in place.

1. To begin, shampoo the hair and gently comb through it, using a wide-toothed comb. Part off about one-and-a-half inches of the front hairline, from recession to recession. This fringe or bang area will remain un-permed. Beginning at the top center, take half-inch triangular sections and wrap every other one on a small-sized perm rod from mid-shaft to scalp. The ends remain free.

2. Secure each rod with stabilizers. For varying degrees of texture, make each section an irregular size.

3. Move to the front sides and continue wrapping sections on small-sized rods. The rods should sit directly on-base. Insert the stabilizers or picks through the bands of adjacent rods to secure the rods in place and keep the bands off of the hair.

4. When both sides are completed, move to the back. Work from the crown down, taking irregularly-sized sections and wrapping every other one. Alternate the stem directions of each wrapped rod for a natural-looking, textural blend.

5. When you reach the nape area, about two-and-a-half inches above the back hairline, take smaller sections than the ones you previously used. Continue wrapping every other one, alternating stem directions. This creates a curlier texture at the nape.

6. Process the alkaline perm according to the manufacturer's directions, rinse, blot and neutralize. Then finish the style as desired. To take maximum advantage of the varied curl patterns, finger-style the finished design, using a diffuser attachment on your dryer.

HAIRLINE PERMS

Hair that has a medium curl pattern is frequently more curly at the nape and front hairline. If the hair is cut into a bob—particularly one that's shorter at the back with diagonal forward sides—the excess curl at the nape interferes with the lines of the cut. The hair below the occipital will stick out farther than intended, and will not fall into the bob line. While "spot" relaxing may provide a solution, the processing time must be precise. A simpler solution that's gentler on hair is to use an acid or alkaline perm solution to soften the growth pattern. The concept is similar to that of the straight perm.

To control uneven curl patterns, Balmer Galindez, of Salon D 'n' B in New York, pre-cuts the hair, leaving it about a half-inch longer than it will be in the final cut. Then he mixes the acid-wave perm solution with one-quarter-ounce of reconstructor/conditioner. The thickened mixture is easy to apply using the following technique:

1. Mix the perm solution and the reconstructor, then section off the nape area with a V-shaped part. Apply the mixture to the curlier nape with a brush.

2. Next take a fine-toothed comb and distribute the product through the hair, working down first, then out. To create direction and make the hair lie flatter, work with the natural growth direction, then against it. After combing the hair downward, part the nape down the center and smooth the hair to the sides, following a diagonal line.

3. If the front hairline is notably curlier than the rest of the hair, also apply the mixture to the front hairline, combing it to lie flat. (Comb the hairline lightly; do not overwork the product into the front hairline.) Then return to the back and continue smoothing it.

4. Depending on the hair's porosity, processing takes from ten to twenty-five minutes for very resistant hair. Periodically recomb the hair so it lies flat; do not walk away and allow processing to continue without combing.

5. When processing is completed, rinse the hair thoroughly and neutralize. Comb the neutralizer into the hair in the same direction that you combed the perm solution so that the hair is "set" in the flatter direction. Wait five minutes, rinse again and complete the cut.

6. If the nape is extremely curly, after the first comb-through of the perm solution mixture, wrap the hair on perm rods to open up the curl. Use the larger-diameter, peach-colored rods. It takes six to eight rods to wrap the entire back nape area. About five minutes before processing is completed, remove the rods, comb

through the hair, rinse, apply the neutralizer and rewrap the rods for the final five minutes. Then remove the rods, rinse the hair and compete the cut.

THE FLAT PERM

Hair that is coarse and straight tends to stick out or "pop up" when the hair is cut very close to the head. This tendency is referred to as the hair being "poppy," and it can destroy the precise lines of a cut. James Christopher Chan of the Hair Resort in Las Vegas, Nevada, created the following technique for his coarse-haired clients, so that he could control growth direction and more easily achieve close-to-the-head looks. The technique works best on hair that is one-and-a-half inches long or shorter.

To use the technique, you'll need a roll of plastic wrap, a comb, a foam perm and a product that allows you to neutralize the perm solution without rinsing, called Pro Ionic Quench. There may be other similar products, and you can try the technique with the perm to which you're accustomed, but the ability to neutralize without rinsing is a definite plus in this instance.

1. Shampoo the hair and treat it with a clarifier to remove any product build-up. Then lightly towel dry the hair.

2. Cut all the hair to the desired length and observe the areas that pop up. These usually occur at the close-cut sides.

3. Apply a foam perm to the "poppy" areas and comb them in the direction of the desired finished style.

4. Carefully compress the permed area with plastic wrap by wrapping it around the head several revolutions before securing it in place. The more tightly you wrap the plastic wrap, the flatter the hair will be. For a better fit, give a half turn to the wrap at the face and/or the occipital.

5. Process the perm according to the manufacturer's directions.

6. When the recommended timing has passed, remove the plastic wrap and immediately apply the Pro Ionic Quench directly to the hair without rinsing out the perm. You are applying the product directly over the thio-based perm. Because it eliminates the rinsing step and completely removes chemical residue from the hair, it allows the hair to be left undisturbed from its flattened pattern.

7. Blot the hair, apply the perm neutralizer and immediately reapply fresh plastic wrap, positioning it tightly around the head as before. After the recommended timing for neutralizing, remove all the plastic wrap and rinse.

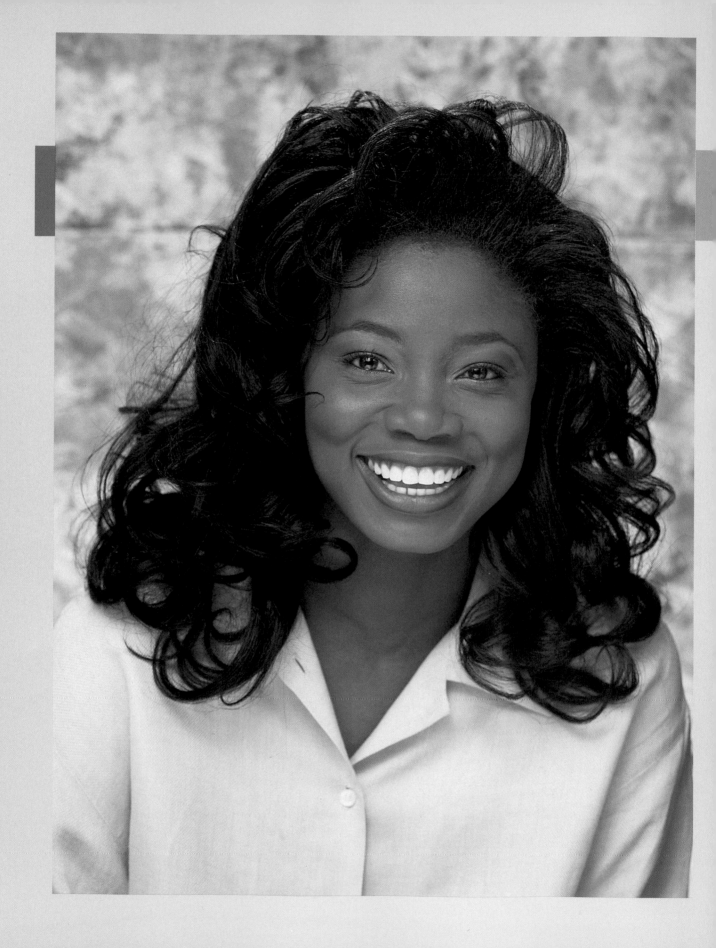

Hair Additions and Extensions

*Hair additions and extensions, known as **weaves** in many African-American communities, allow clients with short or sparse hair to have long, thick hair. **Hair wefts,** which can be attuched in a wide variety of ways, can conceal a bald or thinning patch or a spurse hairline. Individual, prebraided strands can also be attached to the natural hair.*

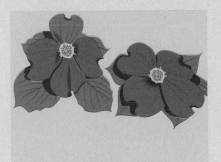

Hair additions come in human and synthetic versions; the choice is a matter of personal preference and economics. Human hair can be shampooed, thermally styled, colored or even permed to match the client's natural hair. It allows maximum versatility, but is also more expensive. Human hair wefts are custom-ordered, using a sample of the client's natural hair.

Synthetic hair comes in a wide variety of hair textures and colors; it is less costly than human hair. Customization is limited because synthetic additions cannot be permed, colored, relaxed or thermally styled; however, they can be purchased in a variety of curl configurations, from straight to extremely curly.

When working with hair additions, pre-plan the placement pattern with the client's goal and the finished style in mind. The simplest placement pattern is to add three to four weft-style additions in the back, evenly spacing them from above the nape hairline to the occipital. In more complex patterns, wefts are added in a circular pattern at the crown or top to conceal a thinning area or they are positioned all throughout the back and the top, to about one inch behind the front hairline.

Analyze the length and condition of the natural hair before proceeding with a hair addition service. The hair should be healthy, without breakage near the scalp, and should be long enough to accommodate or conceal the chosen attachment technique. In complex designs, almost all the natural hair is concealed; in simpler ones, it is incorporated into the hair design.

Any chemical or pressing service should be performed prior to the attachment of the additions. Also, consider your client's lifestyle and willingness to maintain the additions. This will help you decide which hair type and attachment technique to use.

PLACEMENT PATTERNS

As previously noted, placement patterns of hair wefts are based on the desired finished style and the client's goal. While wefts intended to add volume are almost always positioned horizontally—from above the nape to just below the occipital—they may be placed vertically at the sides or top, depending on the desired result.

Horseshoe and completely circular patters are frequently used at the top of the head, as long as the front hairline is parted off and later brushed back to conceal the attachment site. A few small additions can also be added behind the front hairline along a slightly curved line and combed forward to conceal a thinning hairline, to create bangs—or to add fullness. For hairline concealment, use short braided tracks and smaller wefts. (You can cut any weft to the desired width and length.) Individual braids can be added in a bricklay pattern, or any other desired.

Whether wefts are positioned vertically or horizontally, they should be cut or blended in the direction in which they were placed. The simplest way to do this is to divide the head into five sections. Part the hair from ear-to-ear, across the top of the head, to section off the back; then part off the nape. Next divide the front into three equal sections with two horizontal part lines above the temples, just above the recessions. This allows you to easily blend the back horizontally and the top vertically, if that was the placement pattern used and the direction in which hair will lie.

ATTACHMENT TECHNIQUES

Several techniques can be used ito attach hair additions, from a simple bonding method to complex weaving, which requires using thread. The most popular technique requires the creation of on-the-scalp braids, or "tracks," to which hair wefts or additions are attached. Tracks not only mark the path where hair will be attached; they provide a foundation for attachment, because wefts are often sewn on to them. Braided tracks should never be too tight; always perform a complete scalp analysis prior to braiding hair to which additions will be attached. Anytime pin-sized bumps appear around a braid, it is too tight.

CREATING BRAIDS

To create braids, use an underhand technique. In this technique, you create a three-strand swatch and alternately pass each side under the center strand. Take one side or the other with your thumb and forefinger and twist your wrist so that the palm faces upward and the side strand is pulled under the center strand simultaneously. When you create an on-the-scalp braid or cornrow, each time you pass a side strand under the center strand, pick up some of the client's natural hair and add it to the center strand.

Braiding requires practice and patience. If you are not familiar with on- and off-the-scalp braiding techniques, they are described in the following chapter. Hand and wrist movements require that the thumb and forefinger of both hands be used as your working fingers. You will use these fingers to manipulate the hair. Your other fingers are your control fingers. Use them to control the hair, hold it in place and maintain consistent tension as you braid. Each time you pass a side strand under the center strand, transfer it from your working fingers to your control fingers. This results in a new center strand each time.

ADHESIVE OR BONDING METHOD

The bonding method is the simplest attachment technique, in which a weft is attached to the client's natural hair with a latex-based adhesive. While wefts attached with this method are the simplest to remove, they do not last as long as wefts that have been attached using other methods. Wefts may loosen up prematurely if the client is not careful when shampooing and styling, if the client has an oily scalp or if the client uses oil-based hair preparations. This is because the adhesive loosens with oil; the wefts are removed by massaging a mineral-oil product into the attachment site.

Since you cannot use oils or sprays with bonding, the technique is not recommended for hair that will be pressed.

The following technique, from Charlotte Jayne of Garland Drake International, is for adding fullness or volume to fine hair. She recommends that you do not use the technique to add hair that is any longer than twelve-inches, because longer bonded hair will add too much stress to the client's roots. Prior to the service, ask your client about sensitivity to latex; clients who are sensitive should not get extensions that are attached with this method.

Since expensive human hair looks the most natural, you might want to do a "test bond" prior to the service to determine if the client likes the addition and can shampoo and style it correctly. This will avoid disappointment and unnecessary expense on the part of your client.

Human hair should be pre-ordered to match a sample of the client's hair; color, perm or relax it prior to the service if desired. The hair should also be shampooed and dried.

The hairstyle will last four to six weeks, depending on how well the client cares for it and how quickly the hair grows. When it is time to remove the wefts, use an adhesive bond remover or mineral oil. Massage the product into the adhesive to loosen it, and gently slide the weft down the hair shaft.

1. To begin, shampoo and condition the client's hair; then completely dry it. Make certain that no dampness remains.

2. Next section the hair for placement of the hair additions. Placement and the desired number of wefts should have been predetermined, prior to ordering the human hair. Begin by parting off the nape at least an inch above the back hairline. (Fig. 12.1) Make certain the parting is extremely clean, and comb the hair down in natural fall.

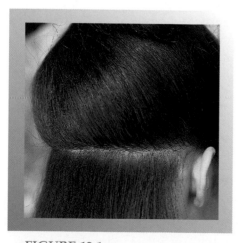

FIGURE 12.1
Part the nape at least an inch above the back hairline.

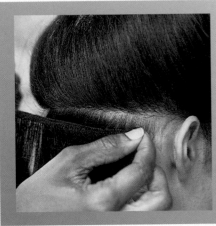
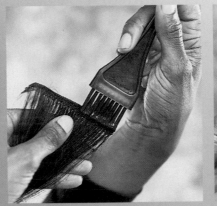
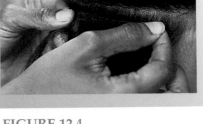

FIGURE 12.2
Hold weft up to parting to determine desired width.

FIGURE 12.3
Apply bonding adhesive to the top of the weft.

FIGURE 12.4
Lightly touch weft to the hair. This will mark where the natural hair should be applied.

3. Hold the weft up to the parting to determine the desired width. You'll want the weft to end at least one-and-a-half inches behind the front hairline on either side. Since this gives you a very wide weft, cut the total desired width in half and apply the weft in two sections. A weft that is wider than four inches does not permit precise control. (Fig. 12.2) (Also, wefts that are narrower reduce the stress on the client's scalp and on the bond, because they weigh less.)

4. Cut the weft to the total desired width; then cut it in half. Apply the bonding adhesive to the top of the weft, on the side where the stitching folds over the hair. Do not shake the product bottle; use the applicator brush to apply the adhesive evenly along the stitching. (Fig. 12.3)

5. Hold the weft up to the hair—from behind the hairline to the center—and lightly touch it to the hair where you will want to apply it. The bonding that transfers during this light touch will mark the path along which you will apply the bond to the natural hair. (Fig. 12.4) This should be at the parting, just below where the scalp shows.

6. Now set the weft aside and apply the bond to the client's natural hair. Make certain that the hair remains straight and smooth as you apply the bond just below the part line. (Fig. 12.5) Remove any bonding product that you get on loose hair and gently smooth any stray hairs.

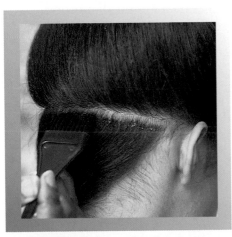
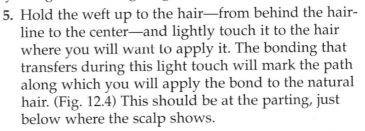

FIGURE 12.5
Apply bond to the client's natural hair.

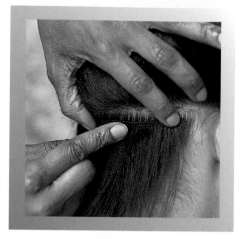

FIGURE 12.6
Press the bond and the natural hair together.

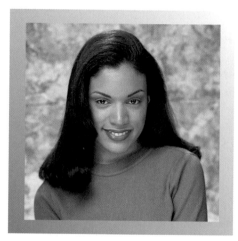

FIGURE 12.7
Finished style, "The adhesive bonding method."

7. Now reapply the bond to the weft, creating a light, second coat, and place the bonded side of the weft against the bond on the client's hair. Firmly press the two together. Use your finger or the end of a comb to do this. Make certain the weft is correctly positioned and firmly set in place, then repeat the procedure with the second half of the weft. (Fig. 12.6) When you position this weft, make certain it is closely aligned with the first one at the center, but does not overlap it.

8. Next move up the head about one-and-a-half inches and part the hair at the point where the second weft will be positioned. (If the client has very thin hair, you can place the wefts closer together as long as there is enough natural hair to which you can attach the wefts.) The positioning of the wefts will also be determined by the desired amount of volume—which is to say, the total number of wefts. Repeat the attachment procedure, applying half the weft to one side and the second half to the opposite side.

9. Continue working up the head until all the wefts have been attached. Generally you will stop just before the crown. If you were to place the weft higher, the natural hair might "split" and reveal the weft's attachment site—particularly if the client's hair is thin. Enough natural hair should remain on top to completely conceal the weft.

10. When all the wefts have been attached, place the client under a hood dryer for at least fifteen minutes to dry the bond. Once the bond has completely dried, inspect your work and proceed with the desired cut. Instruct your client not to shampoo for at least forty-eight hours and demonstrate a gentle shampooing technique that will prevent tugging on wefts.

Reapplication of Wefts

As the natural hair grows out, the wefts will drop down. If the client wants the wefts reattached, apply mineral oil to break down the bonding product, slide the wefts down to remove them, remove the bond residue from the hair with a fine-toothed comb and carefully remove any bond residue from the wefts. Clean the wefts with a toothbrush and detergent to remove any oil, recondition them and make certain they are completely dry. You may now proceed with any desired chemical touch-up services and reapplication of the wefts.

BRAID AND SEW

The braid and sew attachment technique for hair additions is the most commonly used technique, and it can last from six to twelve weeks. If the client's hair is naturally straight, you may need to adjust the additions after six to eight weeks; if it is extremely curly, the curl configuration will "take up" much of the length as the hair grows and the additions will last longer. In this technique, the hair is braided into on-the-scalp cornrows or inverted braids. The braids create a track along which wefts or hair additions are sewn.

This technique is excellent for dense or curly hair; very straight hair may tend to "slip" more easily when you braid it. Hair that is extremely fine will not hold a braid well; a bonding method may work better for this type of hair.

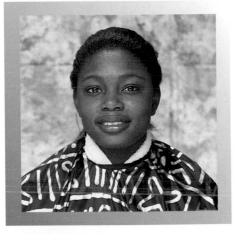

FIGURE 12.8
Before.

Predetermine the placement of the hair additions. In the following technique, a fuller, long, asymmetrical style is desired. For this style, the natural hair should be relaxed, pressed or naturally straight. If the hair is naturally very curly, daily styling will be required to blend the hair to the additions.

To create a simple asymmetrical style, four tracks will be created that move from one side, across the back of the head to the opposite side. The first track is positioned about one-and-a-half inches above the nape hairline. The other three will be evenly spaced up the head and move from a half-inch behind the side hairline, across the back of the head, to the opposite side. Then two vertical tracks will be added on top, toward the heavy side of the asymmetrical part line. These tracks should be spaced so that they are equal distance from the part line, one another, and the side section of your uppermost horizontal track.

The following technique begins with a review of on-the-scalp underbraiding. The four longer braided tracks will be created in two sections. First the hair is braided from the right side to the center; then the hair is braided from the opposite side to the center. Where the braids meet, either join them into a single braid or braid each side to the ends, cross them over the track, then sew them in place to secure.

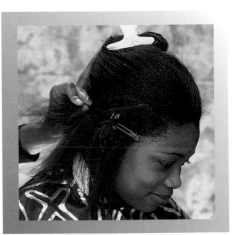

FIGURE 12.9
Following the curve of the head, part the nape.

1. To begin, part the nape with a *U*-shaped parting that follows the curvature of the head. Begin at least one inch above the nape hairline and take a quarter-inch wide part. If hair is fine, make a half-inch parting. (The hair within the part will be braided.) Make certain your parting is clean and that at least a half-inch of hair at the front hairline remains free, to cover the ends of the braid. (Fig. 12.9)

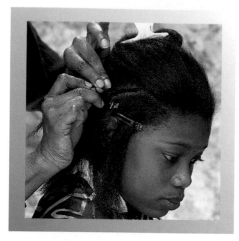

FIGURE 12.10
*Braid by crossing the right strand under
the center strand.*

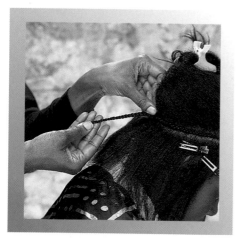

FIGURE 12.11
*Braid the remaining ends and secure into
a mini-ponytail.*

2. Begin at the right side, creating a three-strand, on-the-scalp braid. Divide the hair within the part into three equal sections and begin braiding by crossing the right strand under the center strand. Cross the strand under and transfer the sections with your fingers so that the right strand becomes the new center strand. Then cross the left strand under the new center strand. After crossing the side strands under the center strand two or three times, you may add natural hair to the braid, depending on the technique that you prefer. You can add hair to the center strand each time you cross a side strand under it or add hair to the sides prior to passing them under. The latter technique requires much more expertise and extreme care. (Fig. 12.10)

3. Continue braiding to the center of the back of the head, taking care to maintain consistent tension and follow the curvature of the head. Make certain the braid is clean and neat. When you reach the center back, braid the remaining hair to the ends and temporarily secure into a mini-ponytail. (Fig. 12.11) Then repeat the procedure on the opposite side. When you reach the center, take the ends of the two braids, join them together and divide this new braid into three parts.

4. Braid the new section with three or four crossovers, then secure it with a rubber band. The mini ponytail will be concealed by the weft once it is sewn on to the track.

An alternate technique to finishing off the track is to create a braid support finish. This technique reduces stress on the scalp. To perform it, braid each side of the remaining hair to the ends and secure the ends with a rubber band. Then cross the braid ends over one another onto the track and sew them in place.

5. Next move up the head to the point where the next track will occur and repeat the procedure, beginning with a clean parting. When all four tracks have been completed, move to the top of the head, establish the side part and add the two vertical tracks. They should begin at least an inch behind the front hairline and be about two inches long. (Fig. 12.12)

6. When all the tracks have been completed, attach the wefts to the tracks. Use cotton-covered polyester thread and a straight needle. (If you're accustomed to using a curved needle, use it instead of a straight needle.) (Fig. 12.13) Determine the

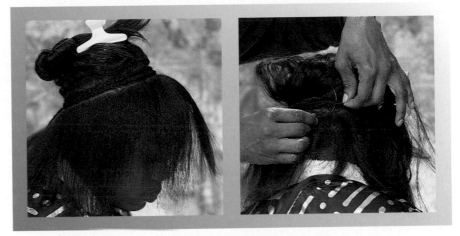

FIGURE 12.12
Add two vertical tracks, at least an inch behind the front hairline and about two inches long.

FIGURE 12.13
Pull the needle through the edge of the weft.

desired width of the weft by holding it up to the track. Then cut the weft to the desired length, leaving about a half-inch extra for safety's sake. Thread the needle, double knot the end and put the needle through the edge of the weft. Secure the knot by creating a loop, then bring the weft up to the first track that you created at the nape.

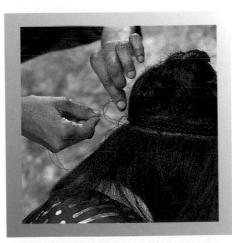

FIGURE 12.14
Pull the needle up until a small loop remains. Then insert the needle through the loop and tighten.

7. Begin sewing the weft onto the track by positioning it at the corner. Pull the needle through the weft and the bottom of the braid as you use your opposite forefinger above the track as a guide. Pull the needle up until a small loop remains; then insert the needle through the loop and pull it tight. Continue sewing along the weft, attaching it to the track, using this lock-stitch technique. (Fig. 12.14)

8. Work consistently and steadily, positioning loops about a quarter-inch apart. When you reach the center, make certain that if you have left a mini-ponytail it is tucked neatly under the weft. Then continue to the opposite side and secure the end by inserting the needle through the loop three or four times. Add a very small drop of speed bond to the knot (not the hair) if desired.

9. Once the first weft is in place, continue sewing the wefts to the tracks in the same order that you created the tracks. When the wefts are securely in place, cut and style the hair as desired.

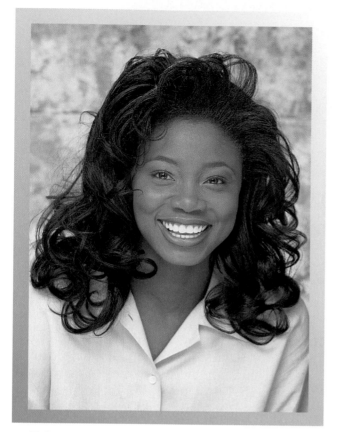

FIGURE 12.15
Finished style, "the braid and sew method."

10. When it is time to re-do the hairstyle, cut the threads across the top and pull them out. Then carefully unbraid the hair and gently brush it out. After shampooing and conditioning the hair, perform a scalp massage as you analyze the scalp and hair. If there are no contraindications, re-create the tracks, positioning in a slightly different place, so that the same hair is not over-stressed.

HAIR WEAVING

Although hair additions are sometimes referred to as "weaves," weaving is a specific attachment technique that utilizes three cords or threads to create a super-secure braid. This braid replaces the French braid or cornrow as the track.

The braids carefully follow the curve of the head so that as the hair grows out, the extensions fall naturally and can be left in place longer. The technique shown here is for the client whose natural hair is at least three inches long in back and at least two inches long at the crown and sides. The tracks are positioned so that the client can wear her hair in an updo. This specific technique comes from Velma Brooks of Dallas, Texas, who first showed it to us; Charlotte Jayne has contributed additional details.

For the weaving method, you need an upright board that will hold three spools of cotton-coated polyester thread or weaving cord. You can purchase one or create your own. The board should hold three spools of thread that run through metal casters, so that the threads remain separated and in place. When you weave, position the board to your side and slightly above the client's head. If you position the board on the right, begin the track on the left side of the client's head.

There are almost as many different methods for weaving as there are professional braiders. In some, you manipulate the hair, not the threads; in others, the threads are manipulated. All require a great deal of practice and patience. However, once you've mastered the art, you can use weaving techniques to give clients who have short, sparse hair or even thinning patches a whole new look. This is because the thread can be used to extend the braid across a thinning area on the head.

1. In this technique, three tracks will be created, upon which the wefts will be attached. (For extra density, you can use a double weft at the middle track.) To begin, create a part that starts just above the right ear, moves to the back where it drops just below the occipital, and continues around the head to behind the left ear. (This placement is for an asymmetrical style; for a symmetrical style, begin and end the track at the same position near both ears.) Create two part lines a half-inch to one-inch apart; the hair in the middle is the hair that will be woven.

2. To begin, pull all three threads out and tie them together. Bring them to the side of the head on which you'll begin. To anchor the first strand, take a quarter-inch strand from the bottom of the parting and wrap all three threads around the strand twice. Then make a loop, pull the knotted end of the threads through the loop and pull it tight. The threads will be positioned near the scalp.

3. Hold the threads and the strand on the scalp with your left forefinger and thumb. Think of the threads as being numbered 1, 2 and 3. With your right hand, reach between the top and middle thread, which are numbered 1 and 2, and pull the strand between the two threads. Then, in sequence, pull thread 2 over the hair, pull thread 3 over the hair and pull thread 1 over the hair. Repeat this sequence two to three times.

4. Now pull the strand up through threads 2 and 3; then pull it down through 2 and 3. Repeat this step three times with the same strand of hair; then pick up a new strand. Repeat the sequence of pulling thread 2, then 3, then 1 over the strand, pull thread 2 to secure the strand, then drop the hair out and continue the pattern with new strands of hair.

5. Continue weaving the braid around the head to the opposite side. Stop when you are between one and a half-inch from the hairline. Then wrap thread 1 over threads 2 and 3, and through a loop to make a knot. Cut threads 1 and 2; thread a large needle onto thread 3 and secure the end with a crisscross lock stitch. Hold the hair down flat to the head as you insert the needle in one direction, then the opposite direction, to create the cross stitch.

6. In this technique, attach the extension before moving up to create the next track. Attach the thread to the extension first, then sew the extension to the braid, inserting the needle from underneath.

7. Position the second track about one inch above the first one, following the same curvature along the head. Create it using the described weaving method.

8. Attach the weft by sewing it to the track, then proceed with the third track. When all the wefts have been sewn onto the hair, cut and style it as desired.

INDIVIDUAL, HIDDEN BRAIDS

While it is more time-consuming, individual strands of hair can be attached to the natural hair, instead of wefts. In this technique, an off-the-scalp, hidden braid is used to hold the attached hair.

The following technique from Charlotte Jayne of Garland Drake International works well for either straight and fine hair or dense and wavy hair because it uses a bonding product to secure the hair addition to the natural hair. The individually attached strands of hair are left free and loose; this technique is not for creating individual cornrows.

Use loose human hair in bulk, or cut small, one-eighth-inch sections from the top of a weft. It is not recommended that you use synthetic hair for this technique, because the fiber will frizz quickly.

Working from about a half-inch above the nape, across the back, strand additions will be added to the natural hair, working from one side to the other. When you move up to the next row, bricklay the attachments so that no braid is directly above the one below it.

1. Begin by making a clean part above the nape, no lower than the occipital bone. Fold the strand of hair over, based on the desired finished length. For thicker, shorter additions, fold the strand in half. For a longer finished look, fold the strand so less than a quarter of the length is on one side of the fold and three-quarters of the length is on the opposite.

2. Pick up a natural strand and position the attachment hair under the natural strand, right at the fold site. Use your left thumb and forefinger to pinch the section where the natural hair meets the attachment strand, then move your forefinger in front of the natural strand. With your right hand, bring the other end of the attachment strand over the forefinger so it is in the center, then close your left thumb over it to hold it there. Repeat bringing the side section over the center section seven times to create an overbraid. Then slide the hair addition up the natural hair strand all the way to the scalp.

3. Place a drop of speed bond at the intersection of the middle and right strands, then cross the natural strand over the bonded area and pinch the resulting braid. Next turn your wrist in order to turn the braid, and apply speed bond to this side. Pinch the braid again and release when the bond has set.

4. Continue the attachment technique, working methodically and carefully from one side to the other. Then move up and take sections of hair in a bricklay pattern.

5. The attachments can be styled as desired for length and fullness. After four to eight weeks, the hair additions should be removed and reattached, if desired.

For more elaborate braiding techniques, read on to the next chapter. After you have completed Chapters 12 and 13, you should be able to combine techniques and even develop your own.

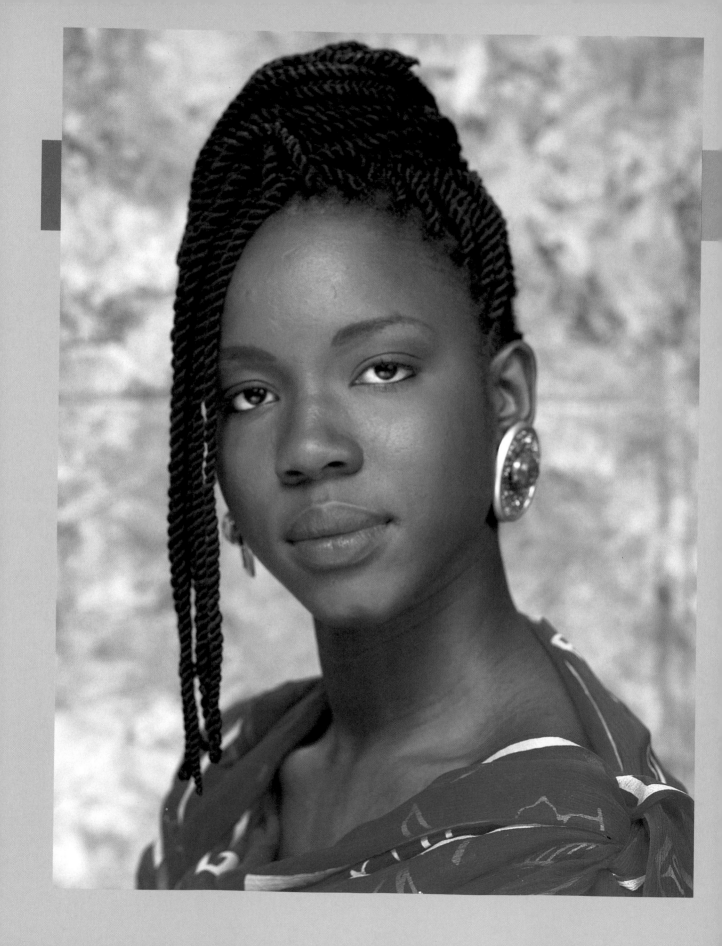

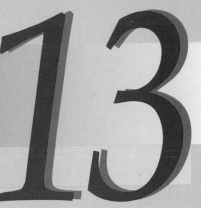

13

Braids and Locks

One of the fastest-growing salon services is braiding, which is tied to the renewed interest in natural hair care and cultural hairstyling.

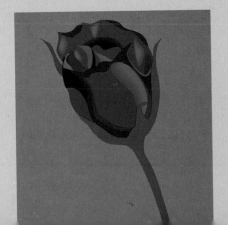

Katherine Jones, the president of the International Braiders Network, has been at the forefront of the movement toward separate licensing for natural hairstylists and shares the following overview of natural hair care and its position in the market today:

> **Natural hair is hair that is free of chemical or thermal applications. Hair that has been chemically or thermally altered can resume its natural state over a period of time; virgin hair has never been touched by either process. This is a new way of thinking for some, because American hairstylists traditionally think of hair that has been thermally altered as still being "virgin."**

NATURAL HAIR CARE AND ITS AFRICAN ORIGINS

Natural hair care is over 4,000 years old and originated in Africa. For centuries, Africans and people of African descent have maintained the natural coil and curl patterns of their hair by braiding, twisting, locking or wrapping it into intricate works of art. Historically, the designs that were created were more than a beautiful hairstyle; they represented an intertwining of identity, spirituality, community, healing and social status.

The African techniques for caring for natural hair have been informally passed down from generation to generation, primarily through oral tradition. While many of the designs and techniques for braiding that are used today are similar to those used in West Africa centuries ago, African Americans have modified them to express their uniquely American experiences. Because those experiences include slavery and racial oppression, hair has come to symbolize something special among African Americans. It is a symbol of their struggle to determine their own, non-European, standards of beauty, cultural identity and pride.

Prior to the 1980s, braiding and natural hair care were a small-scale cottage industry. However, the popularity of natural hairstyles has increased so much that for the first time in the forty centuries that this art form has been practiced, a formal natural-hair-care industry has developed across the nation and abroad. Natural hair care is now considered a profession separate from cosmetology.

THE INTERNATIONAL BRAIDERS NETWORK

With the professionalization of braiding and natural hair care came the formation of the International Braiders Network (IBN). Founded in 1992, the nonprofit organization is committed to the enhancement of braiding and the natural hair care industry. The goals of the organization are threefold. They are:

1. To establish a worldwide network of professional braiders, lockticians and natural hair care specialists.

2. To promote the cultural, historical and technical aspects of braiding, locking and natural hair care.

3. To establish an educational foundation that addresses the needs of natural hair care specialists within the beauty enhancement industry.

The IBN was instrumental in developing and promoting the natural-hair-care license. This separate license was essential because cosmetology laws, which date from the 1930s, mandate that anyone interested in working on hair must attend a cosmetology school and obtain a state license. Natural-hair-care specialists, who do not use chemicals, clearly have different educational needs and goals. The new natural hair care license addresses these needs, and is currently available in New York State. While New York has set the precedent, Washington, D.C., is currently developing a braiding curriculum. Other districts, states and countries are certain to follow. This gives the individual interested in doing hair yet another a new and rewarding career path to follow.

NATURAL HAIR CARE TECHNIQUES

The following descriptions provide you with a basis for creating a few of the most popular braided and locked styles today. This specialized art requires a complete understanding of natural hair care, and, above all, practice and hands-on experience. ÆMDNMØ

CORNROWS

Many techniques can be used to create cornrows. The most common is to create a three-strand, on-the-scalp braid, using an underhand or inverted technique. Shorter hair (about four inches long) can be completely cornrowed in this fashion, so that all the hair on the head is encompassed in custom-designed cornrows. To create braids using hair additions, the same technique is employed, but strands of pre-measured artificial or human hair are incorporated into the cornrow at the scalp, so that longer hairstyles can be achieved. Hair

Note:

In an alternate technique, hair is picked up and added to each strand just before it is passed under the center strand. This technique is also known as inverted or visible French braiding. In another variation that incorporates synthetic hair into cornrows, small strands of synthetic hair are fed into the braid as you work. The ends of the synthetic piece must cross over the ends of the natural hair and be concealed within the braid.

your new center strand before crossing the alternate-side strand underneath it.

4. Complete an entire row in this fashion, then part the next section and begin at the scalp again, creating a three-strand, underhand braid.

Three-Strand Braiding with Hair Additions

To create a long braided style on short hair, add hair additions to the braids.

1. Begin cornrowing by parting off a base in the desired size. Bases can be square, circular, triangular or rectangular. The larger the braids you desire, the larger the base. The smaller the base, the thicker-looking the completed style will be, because it will contain more braids.

2. Divide the base into three equal-sized strands. Then take a pre-measured length of synthetic hair, smooth it and fold it in half, in a U-shape. Position the synthetic strand so that it is centered just above your center strand of natural hair. Join the two sides of the synthetic strand with the two outside strands of natural hair. The center strand of natural hair will show right at the curve of the U-shape.

3. Begin the three-strand, underhand braiding technique by passing one side under the center strand. Then continue underbraiding, alternating the sides as you pass them underneath the center strand.

4. After three to four alternating passes under the center strand, or when you have cornrowed about an inch, redivide the hair into three equal strands. Do this before you run out of natural hair.

5. As you continue braiding, you will now be braiding the synthetic addition all the way to the ends.

Combination Techniques

The technique used for three-strand on-the-scalp braiding can be combined with the technique for adding hair additions. To do this, begin a three-strand braid by joining a folded hair addition to the two sides and alternately crossing the sides under the center strand. Then continue to pick up hair and add it to the center strand as you braid.

Interlocking

In yet another variation, known as interlocking, begin a three-strand underhand braid, add hair to the new center strand and add the synthetic hair to the sides before crossing them under the center strand.

To do this, you must slightly overlap the ends of the natural hair with the synthetic hair and cross the two together under the center strand. Each time you cross an outside strand under the center, add new hair from the scalp to the center strand. Many variations on this technique can be seen in salons across the country; most combine picking up natural hair and incorporating it into the center strand with the hair additions; most also use an underhand braiding technique.

Next add a hair addition to the opposite side strand, cross it under the center strand and pick up hair again, adding it to your new center strand. When you add synthetic or human hair to the sides, overlap the ends prior to crossing under the center strand.

Alternate Attachment Techniques with Hair Additions

Many of the thicker braids seen today are created using hair additions and a two-strand braiding technique. For firm attachment, the natural hair should be at least three inches long. If the natural hair is extremely long, you may not need hair additions, or you may wish to add them to the natural hair create thicker braids.

To attach the artificial hair to the natural hair:

1. Fold the strand of artificial hair in half and hold it at the base of the natural hair.
2. Wrap half of the strand of artificial hair around the base of the natural hair for three to four revolutions.
3. Continue with a two-strand braiding technique.

End Sealing

When braids have been completed and trimmed, the ends are usually heat-sealed to prevent the braid from coming undone. This is only possible when synthetic or artificial hair is used. Synthetic hair is almost always used in braiding techniques because synthetic hair does not "open up" and slip down the natural hair when shampooed. Braided styles created with synthetic hair often last longer, and the hair is less expensive than human hair. In addition, human hair will burn and cannot be neatly heat-sealed at the ends. To seal the ends of synthetic or artificial braids:

1. Trim them evenly. Then hold the ends tightly between your fingertips and hold a match, lighter or other burner to the ends.
2. Roll the singed ends with your fingers until they harden. If desired, curve them upward as you roll.

TYPES OF HAIR

Braids and hair additions are created using human or synthetic hair. Often the choice is made on the basis of cost and weight; however, there are other considerations. Human hair comes in textures from super curly to extremely straight, and it can be permed for a customized curl configuration. Synthetic hair is most often used in braided styles because it comes pre-packaged in long sections that are ideal for braiding. Elaborate, dense styles sometimes require as much as ten pounds of synthetic hair to create. In addition, thick, cotton-like lin fiber is used to create Afrocentric braids, such as the Senegalese twists and corkscrew curls.

Human and synthetic hair can be shampooed; lin fiber cannot; therefore, styles created with lin require daily cleansing of the scalp with an antiseptic. Lin fiber and synthetic hair come in pre-packaged bundles, and your supplier can guide you as to about how many are required to create a specific style.

SENEGALESE TWISTS

Senegalese twists have their origin in West Africa. These braids are created using thick strands of lin fiber and a two-strand braiding technique. Pre-plan the final look to determine how much hair you will need. This will be determined by the length of the desired braids and the size of the partings. The smaller the partings, the more braids you will create.

Each fiber strand should be about thirty to thirty-six inches long, accounting for length lost from braiding, and at least a half-inch to one inch in diameter. Pre-purchase the fiber and divide it into as many strands as you want braids in advance of the service.

To control the natural hair and the fiber strand, you may want to slick the hair with gel. Although each fiber strand will be relatively thick, braiding it tightly will create a braid that is thicker than a normal cornrowed braid but not as thick as you might anticipate. Practice braiding the twists tightly to gain an understanding of how thick a strand of hair fiber you need to create the desired final effect.

1. Begin by selecting lin fiber that matches the client's in color and texture and separate the fiber into thick, individual strands. For shoulder-brushing braids, the fiber strand should be about thirty inches long.

2. Part a section of the client's hair at the temple hairline. The smaller the section, the more braids you will have to create for the finished design and the fuller it will be. (Fig. 13.7) For fewer, more obvious braids, larger partings may be more desirable. Slick the ends of the natural hair for extra control.

3. Fold the strand of lin fiber in half. Hold the folded center at the base of your parting, right above the natural hair. The two sides of the fiber strand should

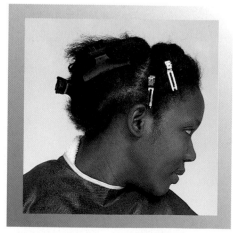

FIGURE 13.7
Part hair at temple hairline.

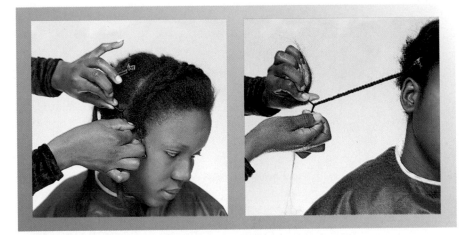

FIGURE 13.8
Wrap half of the hair fiber three to four revolutions around the natural hair.

FIGURE 13.9
Twist one strand over the other to create a tight braid.

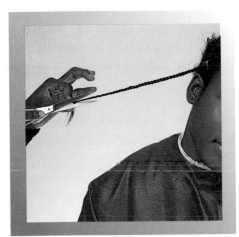

FIGURE 13.10
Seal the ends in the predetermined fashion.

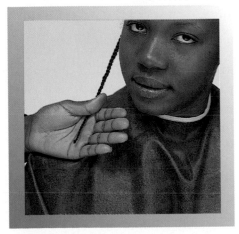

FIGURE 13.11
Finished sealed ends.

hang down on either side of the natural hair. Then wrap half of the hair fiber three to four revolutions around the natural hair. Hold the natural hair and the center point of the fiber strand tightly as you wrap half of the fiber strand firmly around the natural hair. (Fig. 13.8)

4. Make certain the attachment site looks smooth and natural. Next begin creating a two-strand braid with the fiber strand. If natural hair remains, incorporate it into one side of the fiber strand or the other as you cross the two strands over one another until there is no natural hair left. Roll the hair between your fingers, then twist one strand over the other to create a neat, tight braid. (Fig. 13.9)

5. Continue crossing the strands over one another to the end. Hold the hair firmly and tightly as you braid to create a smooth, natural-looking braid. When you reach the ends, seal them in the desired fashion, depending on the finished style. (Fig. 13.10) You can heat seal the ends, add a decorative shell before sealing the ends or tie the ends with string and cut off the excess string. (Fig. 13.11)

6. Continue creating twists throughout the hair, working back from the temple, across the back to the opposite side. Then complete the sections below and above the center strip. You may wish to custom design braids at the top front to move forward or off the face. When all the hair has been braided into Senegalese twists, the

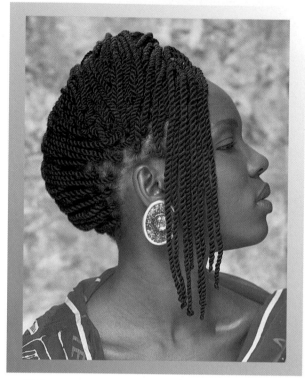

FIGURE 13.12
Finished style, "Senegalese twist."

twists can be further designed by arranging them around the head and sewing them in place.

Corkscrew Curls

Corkscrew curls are created using a similar technique as that used to create Senegalese twists. Because corkscrew curls are intended to be large and thick, larger-than-normal partings are used, in square, triangular or rectangular shapes. The partings become part of the finished design.

To create the corkscrew effect, attach a section of cord or thread that is twice as long as the strands of hair fiber to the base and wrap it around the fibers. Thread in any color or thickness can be used, adding to the decorative appeal and customization of the design. For a more sophisticated look, try using thick metallic thread. Avoid elastic threads; they are difficult to control and will result in uneven bunching of the finished curl.

1. Begin at the nape by taking a one-inch square parting. For variations, use triangular or rectangular partings that are larger or smaller in size.

2. Attach the cord to the base of the hair by wrapping one end several revolutions around the base of the natural hair. Then tie the cord firmly in place.

3. Take a thick strand (at least a half-inch in diameter) of hair fiber that is half as long as the thread, fold in half and position the center of the strand at the base, where the thread is tied. Position the fiber strand vertically. Then tie the fiber strand in place securely with the thread.

4. Fold the half of the hair fiber that moves upward down, over the natural hair and the other half of the fiber strand. Spread it out to cover all the natural hair and the other half of the fiber strand. Lin fiber is thick and cotton-like enough to do this easily.

5. Then take the cord in one hand and the single section of hair in the other. Twist the lin fiber counterclockwise as you wrap the cord or thread in a clockwise direction. Begin to wrap the thread around the hair at an angle. As you pull the thread toward you, use the opposite hand to push the strand of lin upward, toward the scalp.

6. Continue wrapping the thread or cord around the strand. Maintain the same angle each time and make certain that the thread crosses the hair at regular intervals. Use consistent tension each time you wrap the thread around the hair, and push the hair up to the same degree each time to create an even corkscrew effect. Make certain that the hair is smooth each time you wrap the thread around it.

7. Work methodically and quickly to the bottom of the braid, then wrap the thread around the braid two or three revolutions and tie it in place. Cut off any excess thread or hair fiber.

8. Work across the back of the head, creating corkscrew curls at the nape, then move up the head, part a new row and begin again. Maintain consistent sized and shaped partings as you complete the entire head in this manner. When you reach the top, you may want to direct the braids to one side or the other, depending on the finished style. The corkscrew curls can be left to hang free or wrapped up to create yet another design.

GODDESS BRAIDS

Technically, a goddess braid is larger than usual and is an inverted braid or cornrow. Some goddess styles use several large braids; others take about several pounds of hair to create. Human hair is not used to create goddess braids because of the weight and the prohibitive cost.

With the goddess technique, part long, somewhat wide sections of hair based on a pre-planned design. As you braid across the curve of the head, you will incorporate the natural hair into the braid.

The braids can move from one side across to the center back (along a slight diagonal), from the perimeter up to the center top or in any direction desired. Usually the natural and synthetic hair is braided on-the-scalp to a predetermined point, then the synthetic addition is braided all the way to the ends. When the entire head is completed, the free-hanging braids are wrapped up on top of the head into a pre-planned design. In a variation, vertical goddess braids can be allowed to hang free or be cut into a bob.

1. Begin by parting the hair. The width of the parting and amount of synthetic hair used will determine the size of the braid. (Fig. 13.14) Since goddess braids are generally used to create a final updo, take a vertical section. In this instance, it will be about five inches wide.

2. Split the section vertically in half and pull out a piece of hair at the end, closest to the scalp, where you will begin attaching the synthetic hair. (Fig. 13.15)

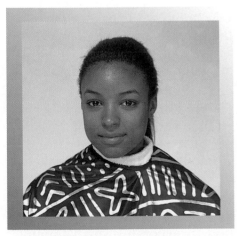

FIGURE 13.13
Before.

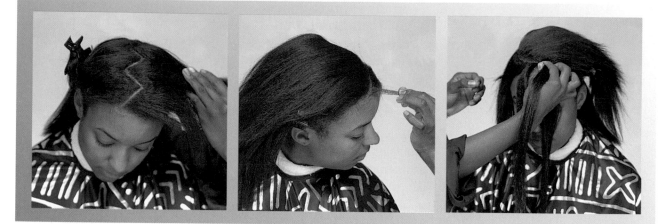

FIGURE 13.14
Part the hair.

FIGURE 13.15
Pull out a piece of hair at the end.

FIGURE 13.16
Drape one synthetic strand over the other so that they cross at the center.

3. Take two synthetic strands or hair extensions in the predetermined length and fold both evenly in half, in a *U*-shape, or horseshoe. Drape the strands over one another so they cross at the center of the horseshoe. (Fig. 13.16) You will have four strands hanging down, which you will now incorporate into three strands.

4. Hold the strands at the point where they loop over one another, bring one strand over to act as your center strand and equally redistribute another strand between the other two to create your two side sections. The synthetic hair is now divided into three sections.

5. Bring the synthetic hair to the base of the small section of natural hair that you previously pulled out. Position the apex of the synthetic strand at the base of the natural strand and fold the natural hair over the synthetic hair to cover the center section. Make certain that the ends of the natural hair will be concealed within the braid when you begin braiding.

6. Begin braiding, using a three-strand underhand technique. (Fig. 13.17) Each time you cross one of the sides under the center strand, pick up some of the natural hair and incorporate it into the center strand. Make certain that the natural hair is concealed by the center strand and does not show on the surface.

7. Many braiders use an overhand technique. To do this, begin with a side section, incorporate a small amount of natural hair into it and bring it over the center section. Then take the opposite side, pick up natural hair

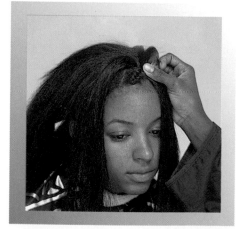

FIGURE 13.17
Begin braiding, using a three-strand, underhand technique.

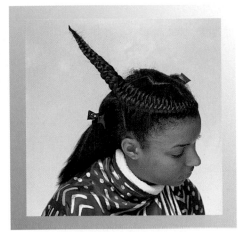

FIGURE 13.18
Braid the hair to the ends.

with it and bring it over the center strand. Continue in this manner, bringing side sections over the center section of the braid. Because the five-inch section was divided vertically in half, it is simple to incorporate natural hair from the appropriate side.

8. Work almost to the center back, or any other pre-determined stopping point. Then braid the hair to the ends. (Fig. 13.18)

9. Move up the head, take another long, five-inch wide parting and continue the braiding technique. As you move up the head, these partings will become more steeply curved for an asymmetrical design. When one half of the head is completed, move to the opposite side and braid it, based on a predetermined design. Trim and singe the ends of the braids. At the point where free-hanging braids meet one another, wrap them up or around the head in a pre-planned design.

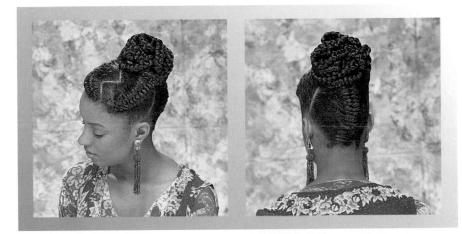

FIGURE 13.19
Finished style, "goddess braids."

FIGURE 13.20
Finished style, back view.

CASAMA BRAIDS

Casamas are created by using individual partings and braids that are larger in size than box braids or single braids. To braid them, use the attachment technique for the Senegalese twists and continuing with three-strand braiding. The stitch of the braid itself is very tight, which allows the braid to curve when finished. The technique begins at the nape, where square, triangular or rectangular partings are taken in any size desired. For the typical style, squares are one-half to one-inch square. The first two or three rows from the nape up can be horizontal; when you reach the top, preplan your design based on whether an asymmetrical look is desired or not. If it is, cre-

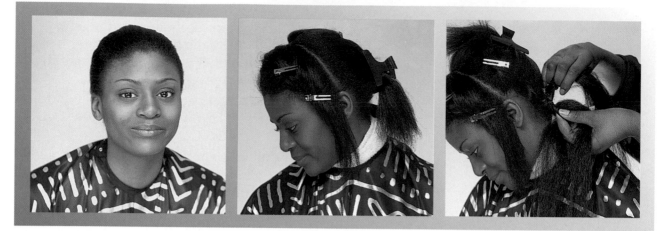

FIGURE 13.21
Before.

FIGURE 13.22
Part hair at the temple with a vertical part.

FIGURE 13.23
Position the center of the strand at the base of the parting. Wrap around the base of the parted natural hair.

ate a side part and plan to create braids that begin at the part line and move across the top of the head. This means the partings will follow an angled line and will not be perfectly horizontal at the top.

When the entire head is completed in the desired fashion, the free-hanging braids are singed with a burner.

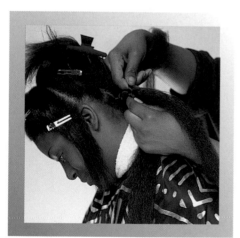

FIGURE 13.24
Divide the hair into three sections and begin three-strand braiding.

1. Begin by parting at the template with a vertical part. Base the depth on the desired finished look. (Fig. 13.22) Now take square, triangular or rectangular sections, beginning at the side.

2. Take a strand of synthetic hair in a predetermined length and fold it in half. Position the center of the strand at the base of the parting and wrap one half three or four revolutions around the base of the parted natural hair. (Fig. 13.23)

3. Immediately divide the hair into three sections, with the natural hair encompassed into the center section. Make certain that the natural hair is concealed under the section before you begin three-strand braiding. (Fig. 13.24)

4. Braid the hair from scalp to ends, using an underhand or inverted technique. Each time you pass a side strand under the center strand, bring the center strand over tightly, so that the side strand becomes the new center strand. Then pass the alternate side strand under this one.

5. When you reach the ends, pull out a long, small section of hair, wrap it around the braid several times, knot it and repeat

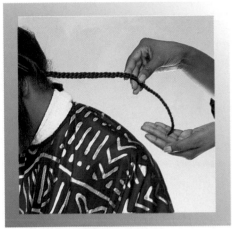

FIGURE 13.25
Seal the ends.

wrapping and knotting. This holds the tight braid in place and allows it to curve. Then continue to the next parting and repeat the entire procedure. Move up the head, taking partings according to the pre-planned design.

6. When the entire head is completed, you can heat-seal the ends or decoratively tied thread. (Fig. 13.25)

Individual Braids

Box braids are simply individual braids of any size that are left to hang free; the braids themselves become the style. They can be created on long, natural hair or by attaching human or synthetic hair to the base of each parting and creating a three-strand braid. Synthetic hair can be burned at the ends.

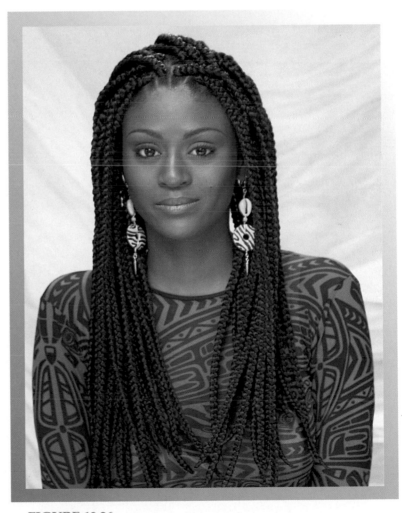

FIGURE 13.26
Finished style, "casama braids."

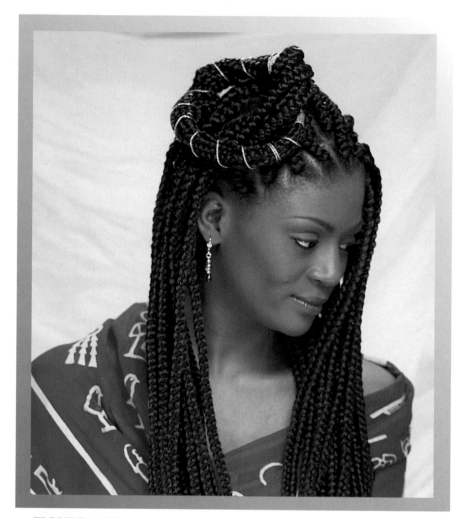

FIGURE 13.27
Elegant style, casama braids.

When creating box braids, make certain the base of the braid is not so tight that potential breakage can result. If you see pinhead-sized bumps on the scalp, the braid is too tight. You can use the goddess technique to create free-hanging box braids and cut them into a bob. Many other braiding techniques can be combined for various end results, based on the artist's skill and vision.

HAIRLOCKING

Hairlocking is the process that occurs when coily hair is allowed to develop in its natural state without the use of combs, heat or chemicals. Lockticians distinguish between curl and coil, noting that coiling describes the interaction between strands of hair. The more revolutions in a single strand, the faster the hair will coil and lock.

Nekhena Evans, a Brooklyn-based locktician and the author of "Everything You Need to Know About Hairlocking," provided the following information on the history of locks, their spiritual and cultural significance and the technique for creating them today.

In most Aboriginal societies, locked hair is regarded as sign of religious consecration or a favor bestowed upon an individual by God. The "chosen" person inherits a spiritual vocation to serve as a messiah, priestess, diviner, prophet, disciple or sadhu (holy person). For example, in the Yoruba religion, devotees of DaDa are identified by their locked hair; in Ghana, only priestesses wear their hair in locked styles. Historically, hairlocking is a sacred hairstyle that has also been a symbolic declaration of rebirth.

Since antiquity, tribes in Africa from Egypt, to Nubia, to Cush, have celebrated the sanctity of the head. The concept of hair as one's "crowning glory" is derived from this spiritual perspective. Perceived as sacred and as the seat of spiritual power, hair was not merely an extension of the head, but a spiritual center to be groomed, adorned and fashioned with purpose. At the very heart of the ancient African hair tradition is the seed for the unique contributions that African Americans have made to the field of natural hair care. To understand the historical role hair has played in African culture is to understand African-American standards for both hair and beauty.

In Biblical times, the Nazarites vowed to wear their hair in locks as a visible sign of their consecration to the Lord. According to the law of the Nazarite in *Numbers* 6:5: "All the days of the vow of his separation shall no razor come upon his head: until the days be fulfilled in which he separateth himself unto the Lord, he shall be holy and shall let the locks of his hair of his head grow." Jesus Christ was a Nazarite.

Locks were important in other parts of the world as well. In the Caribbean, Rastafarians began wearing locks in adherence to the Priestly Code in *Leviticus*. *Leviticus* 21:5 says: "They shall not make baldness upon their head, neither shall they shave off the corner of their beard, nor make any cuttings in their flesh." In India, the Sadhus or Holy Men wear their hair in locks as part of their spiritual vows.

In the spiritual tradition, the hair locks on its own, instinctively and naturally. It has been reported that locks have emerged instantaneously in an ecstatic religious experience.

Historically, hairlocking reflected sociocultural denominations, communicating the identity of the wearer. Events such as tribal rites of passage for warriors, marriage, birth and death were indicated by the wearing of locks. In Africa today, lock wearing continues to communicate specific information.

For cultural purposes, "African" locks are intentionally cultivated. They are formed by parting the hair and individually palm rolling each section with clay and oil. The African clays of choice come in a variety of shades; oils are derived from the palm nut or other types of nuts, or from animal fat. Today people choose to lock their hair for cultural, spiritual or aesthetic reasons. The term *dreadlocks* has been improperly placed on this beautiful process of allowing the hair to grow naturally, but as the art of hairlocking grows, so, too, will respect for and understanding of this ancient tradition.

African Lock Cultivation

Coily hair will lock on its own without cultivation because of the hair's natural ability to intertwine. When left to its own devices—and the elements—coily hair transforms into what most of us know as Rastafarian locks. Even if hair is straight, it can mat to form individual locks; however, it cannot form true, coiled locks.

Cultivated locks that are intentionally guided through the natural process of locking are known as African locks. There are five primary ways to create them. Twisting, braiding and wrapping coily hair will all result in hair locks if the hair is left undisturbed over a period of time. Some lockticians use a comb to lift sections of hair and twist them into locks.

In the salon, the preferred and most effective technique is palm rolling. This method is also gentlest on the hair as it guides it through the four natural stages of hair locking. Palm rolling takes advantage of the hair's natural ability to coil.

Palm-Rolled Locks

When consulting with the client who is considering locks, it is important to stress that once the hair is completely locked, the locks can only be removed by cutting them off. The client who has had any chemical service has rearranged the hair's natural structure; therefore, the hair must be grown out before it can be cultivated by palm rolling.

After the initial service, the locks are maintained during subsequent services. The hair locks in progressive stages, which take six months to a year to complete. During the first few months, the client should return to you every four to six weeks to have the locks cleaned, conditioned and re-rolled. After the hair locks into solid, compacted coils, it can be shampooed regularly; once every two weeks is most common. Then the locks can be worn for years with regular maintenance. They should be kept clean and lint-free, and be moistened with a light non-petroleum-based oil. Heavy oils and gels should be avoided.

Almost any length hair can be palm rolled; about six inches is the ideal length. If the hair is shorter, you may have to manipulate the locks by finger rolling them instead of palm rolling them.

To prepare for palm rolling, you'll need a spray bottle of water, a rattail comb, clips for holding the hair and a light pomade or light, alcohol-free gel.

1. To begin, shampoo and condition the hair. Then towel blot the hair, squeezing out excess moisture so that the hair is damp but not wet.

2. Next part the hair in horizontal rows from the nape all the way to the front hairline. Then divide the first horizontal row at the nape into equal-sized subsections. The subsections can be square, circular, triangular or rectangular; the size of the individual sections and their shape depends on the client's desired finished look. Before palm rolling, use the hair clips to hold the hair around the subsection out of the way.

3. Beginning at the nape on the far right side, take the hair within the first subsection and lightly apply a pinch of gel, using your right forefinger and thumb. Then pinch the hair near the scalp and twist it one full clockwise revolution. (If you are left-handed, use your left hand to pinch the hair, but always turn it clockwise.)

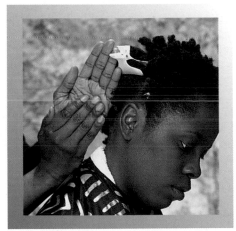

FIGURE 13.28
Pass the hair from your right hand to your left.

4. With one smooth motion, pass the hair from your right hand to your left hand, tuck the hair into the recession near the thumb and fold your thumb down to hold the hair in place. Position your left hand behind your right hand so that the left fingertips are at the right wrist. Slide your right hand back while simultaneously sliding the left hand forward. (Fig. 13.28)

5. When the hair is between your palms, pull out your thumb so that the hair is rolled between your palms. When the fingertips of your right hand are near the left-hand wrist, fold your thumb back down to recapture the hair.

6. So that the hair is always rolled in a clockwise direction, reposition the left hand behind the right hand and repeat the palm rolling technique. Each time you roll the hair, move progressively down the hair shaft. When you reach the ends, place the lock down neatly and begin again with the adjacent subsection.

7. When each subsection in the first horizontal row has been completed, move up to the next horizontal row and subdivide it as before. If you rolled the previous subsections from right to left, this time work from left to right. Continue this pattern all the way to the crown. As you work up the head, include the side sections. Always maintain a consistent degree of

moisture by using the spray bottle as needed. Also, apply the same amount of gel to each subsection.

8. When you reach the crown, continue palm rolling subsections, directing them to move toward the back. When you reach the top of the head, move around the client to accommodate the desired finished style. If the client wants the front individualized, for instance, if a few sections are to move onto the forehead, reposition yourself in front of the client to palm roll these subsections.

9. When all the hair has been palm rolled, place the client under a hood dryer set on low heat. Dry the hair completely, but no more than necessary.

10. When the hair is completely dry, finish the style by applying a light oil to add sheen.

11. For the first three months, the client should come back every four weeks to have the locks cleaned and re-rolled. It is extremely important to remove any embedded lint during this stage, before the hair compresses into tight locks. Remove lint with a small fine toothbrush. If it is necessary to brush out the lock or open it up and re-roll it to do this, assure the client that this will not disturb the locking process. Experienced locticians have noted that once hair begins to coil and lock, re-rolled locks will return to their precise stage of development.

HOME CARE FOR BRAIDS AND LOCKED STYLES

Locks and braids can be cleaned in a similar fashion. Instruct the client to use following technique:

Apply shampoo directly to the scalp and perform an intense scalp massage, without disturbing the hair locks. After massaging, place a stocking cap or mesh scarf over the head and rinse the hair for at least five minutes, until the water runs clear. Then, perform a second washing by applying shampoo directly over the cap and lightly massaging the scalp again. Rinse the hair for at least five more minutes, then allow the locks to dry with the cap left in place.

The client should sit under a dryer that is set on low heat until the hair is dry. (Wait until the hair has cooled before removing the stocking cap.) Then apply a light oil to the locks to restore moisture.

When locks have reached the "adult" stage, that is, when they become compressed locks, they can be deep-cleaned by applying a lemon rinse to the dry hair. Mix two parts water and one part fresh squeezed lemon juice, and pour the mixture into a spray bottle. Set the spray bottle adjustment to create a stream, not a mist, and spritz each lock as you gently manipulate it. Then proceed with shampooing, as previously described.

HOME CARE FOR BRAIDED STYLES THAT USE DIFFERENT TYPES OF HAIR

Synthetic and human hair can be shampooed in the same manner as natural locks are; most braiders recommend shampooing just once every two weeks. Braids should be shampooed lightly and gently, using a wax-free shampoo that was specifically formulated for braids. Leave-in conditioners should be used sparingly.

After shampooing, braids can be carefully towel dried by patting. Human hair wefts can be partially dried under a hood dryer. After drying braids, a light amount of braid oil should be sprayed directly onto the braids. The scalp should also be oiled as needed, if done sparingly.

Lin fiber should not be washed. If the client has a style that uses lin fiber, she should carefully clean the scalp each day, using a cotton ball and witch hazel or an antiseptic. After the scalp between each braid has been cleaned, the braids can be lightly oiled.

Since haircolor is one of the fastest-growing services in all markets, you'll not only be coloring more brunettes in the future; you'll frequently face decisions about how to perform double-chemical services safely. Your biggest challenge: How to safely color hair of all types that has been permed or relaxed. The "graying of America," or aging of the population, will also create an increased demand for expertise in gray coverage.

This chapter and the one that follows address advanced techniques essential for becoming a multinational, multicultural haircolorist, whose abilities know no boarders. As an advanced cosmetologist, you are already familiar with color theory, the principles of the color wheel and proper color selection. If not, refresh your memory by referring back to an introductory haircolor textbook or by taking a color class to brush up on haircolor basics.

COLOR CHEMISTRY BY CATEGORY

Natural pigment or melanin found in the cortex layer of the hair determines its natural color. Gray is simply absence of pigment. When changing the hair's color with a **permanent product or oxidative tint,** the product penetrates the cuticle and deposits artificial color in the cortex. Oxidation occurs when the ammonia in the haircolor reacts with the hydrogen peroxide in the developer.

Permanent colors lighten the natural hair by breaking the melanin down into smaller particles first, just as lighteners do. The degree of lightening depends on the oxidizing agent (usually hydrogen peroxide), its strength and the amount of time it is left on the hair. Then the artificial-color molecules penetrate the cuticle to the cortex and enlarge during oxidation to become trapped there. Since this requires a chemical change in the hair, the hair's porosity, condition and previous chemical treatments are essential parts of the equation for safely and correctly coloring any hair type.

Metallic dyes and vegetable colors, such as henna, are classified as permanent haircolors because, over time, with repeated use, they build up on the hair shaft, penetrate the hair fiber and either attach to the bonds in the hair or actually form bonds via a reaction between the sulfur in keratin and the metallic salts.

Semi-permanent colors have color molecules that are small enough to penetrate the cuticle, but they do not penetrate farther, nor do they anchor themselves in the cortex. For this reason semi-permanent colors fade gradually, over a four to six week period.

Temporary colors simply coat the cuticle with color, which is removed with a single shampoo. Because of the molecular weight of the dye molecules in temporary haircolor products—and the absence of a chemical reaction—they do not penetrate to the cortex.

A somewhat new color category that combines the benefits of temporary and semi-permanent colors has several names: **demi-permanent;** no-lift; long-lasting semi-permanent; no-ammonia; no-peroxide and so forth. These colors do not lift color, but deposit only. However, they last longer than traditional semi-permanent colors due to their unique chemistry. This makes them ideal for clients who have permed or relaxed hair. (Most of these colors use some type of developer, which despite its name does contain a small amount of hydrogen peroxide.)

CONTRIBUTING PIGMENT

Haircolor products come with easy-to-use charts and swatches, which assist you in color selection. They rely on the level system, which measures depth of color (darkness or lightness) and the color's tonality (warmth or coolness). Any level of color can be warm, cool or neutral.

Two factors that demand special attention are the color swatches and the role of contributing pigment.

Color swatches are almost always created by coloring hair that has been de-pigmented or is devoid of color. As a result, the "true color" of the product is displayed, but it has little relationship to how that color product will actually look on your client's hair. When performing a color consultation, it is simpler to have the client show you photos of the colors she likes. This way she will not unrealistically expect her newly colored hair to look precisely like the color swatch.

The primary reason the same product will always look different on a particular client is because of her contributing pigment, or natural haircolor. (Porosity, the hair's condition, product usage, sun exposure and other factors also play a role.) Contributing pigment varies from individual to individual, and even varies along the hair shaft of an individual.

The following information on using contributing pigment to make a color decision comes from Richard Cardone, a Clairol haircolor educator who has over twenty years of experience coloring hair and who owns Richard Cardone Hair Designers and Color Specialists in Pittsburgh, Pennsylvania.

Contributing pigment must always be considered when coloring hair, particularly if you want to lighten the natural color by more than two levels. Hair that is naturally dark, from Level 1 to Level 3,

◆ Use a brightener prior to applying a demi-permanent color to break down the compact cuticle. Mix a mild brightener with 10 volume developer, process for ten to fifteen minutes with no heat, rinse, then apply the desired demi-permanent shade.

◆ As an option to using a brightener, pre-soften the hair with an oil lightener. If you pre-soften with a product that requires the addition of activators, use one activator or none. Rake the product through the hair in broad streaks, process for ten to fifteen minutes without heat and rinse. This breaks the base and creates porosity in the hair. You can then continue with a semi-permanent shade to add a casting or tone of red, plum or gold. Semi-permanents are excellent for this purpose if true lifting is not desired.

◆ If hair is dark in color and resistant—and the desired effect is a change in levels—pre-lighten the hair first. Pre-lighten only to the level necessary to achieve the desired results. If hair is dark brown and true ash blonde is the desired result, you must pre-lighten to the gold stage. Remember, this technique is primarily for virgin hair. Even if hair has been permed using a one-step process, it will be porous enough that pre-lightening may not be required, depending on desired level of the final result.

◆ Hair that has medium curl or an extreme-curl pattern presents more of a control challenge. It is much simpler to weave out sections of straight hair for foil highlighting than it is to weave super-curly hair. However, freeform techniques, such as painting-on color, make highlighting very curly hair simple.

If hair is very curly or has had previous chemical treatments, it is imperative that you perform porosity and elasticity tests prior to coloring the hair. As a general rule, the finer or more porous the hair, the more quickly it reacts to any chemical process, including coloring.

SELECTING A COLOR CATEGORY

If you have performed a thorough, analysis-based consultation, selecting the type of color product to use is simplified. Permanent color allows dramatic changes because it can lighten and darken a wide range of natural haircolors. Extremely dark level 1 or 2 natural colors may require double-processing if the desired result is level 7 through 10. Permanent oxidizing tints remain the best option for complete gray coverage and for clients who want their color to last as long as possible.

Semi and demi-permanent color products are best for clients who are "trying on" color for the first time or whose hair has had previ-

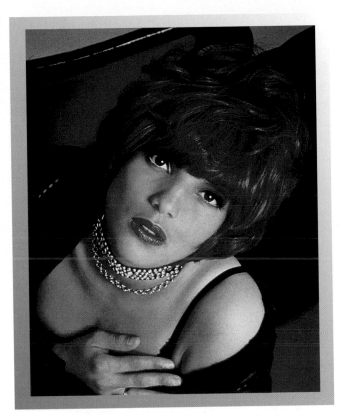

FIGURE 14.2
Relaxed hair with semi-permanent color. Hair: Barbara Marshall and Rhonda Hicks for Professional Results International, Inc. and Emuges by Hair Station USA; Makeup: David Pollard; Photo: George Wong.

ous chemical services, including perms and relaxers. They're also ideal for special effects coloring or adding lowlights. Keep in mind that you cannot lighten hair with these products; therefore, contributing pigment and the desired final results are vital to consider when determining color limitations. These products can be used on naturally dark-colored hair for gray coverage if lift is not desired. (Be certain to mix a neutral into your formula to combat brassiness if hair is not completely gray.)

Temporary color products are safe and gentle for all hair types and are excellent for introducing clients to color. However, if the natural hair is extremely dark and has a compact cuticle, do not expect to see a highly visible difference unless the particular product is heat-activated or you can make it semi-permanent by adding a low volume of hydrogen peroxide. (Often, these are polymer colors that are classified by purists as semi-permanent.) With polymer colors, you can achieve fashion shades of grape, violet and red on the darkest of natural colors. However, these fashion shades will not come out with one shampoo, so make certain your client wants dramatic color results before proceeding.

PREVIOUS SERVICE CONSIDERATIONS

Previous chemical services that have been performed on hair limit your choice of color products. If hair has had a previous chemical treatment, always perform a porosity test and a strand test before using permanent hair color.

Permanent color products can be used on relaxed hair a week after the relaxing service, but they are generally not recommended for hair that has been permed using a two-step process because the hair has already been exposed to drying thio-based chemicals. Excessive drying and related problems may result. Check the hair's condition and perform a strand test before using a permanent color on hair that has been permed using a two-step process.

When using permanent color on relaxed hair, use lower volumes of developer whenever possible. If a client wants to lift her color more than two levels, it will be necessary to perform a double

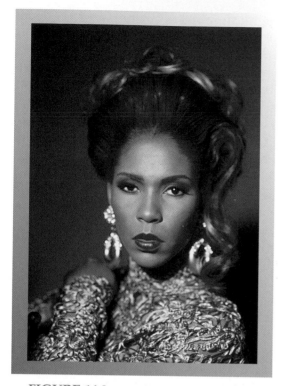

FIGURE 14.3
Cut, color and style. Hair: Barbara Marshall and Rhonda Hicks for Professional Results International, Inc. and Emages by Hair Station USA; Makeup: David Pollard; Photo: George Wong.

process by first decolorizing hair using a lightener, then depositing the desired shade in a second step. It is never recommended that you use a double-process color technique on relaxed hair or hair that has had a two-step perm.

Even if hair has had a single-step perm, each time the hair's bonds are broken and reformed, a few remain broken. Double processing compounds this problem, and hair that has been repeatedly permed and decolorized takes on a spaghetti-like look and feel because too many bonds remain broken.

When hair is unevenly porous due to previous chemical treatments, you can even out porosity with a filler, but performing a strand test remains essential. This will predict uneven color results, which you may be able to compensate for by varying the formulation or volumes of peroxide for different areas of the head.

Keep in mind, the more chemical stress, the more likely it is that you will compromise the hair's condition. If your initial consultation indicates that a client is interested in haircolor and a second chemical service, you can plan for both in advance by using gentler relaxers, mild perms or a two-step perming technique without a booster. Then suggest conditioning and moisturizing treatments prior to the single-step color service, which should take place a week later if a permanent haircolor is used.

Semi-permanent, no-lift, or demi-permanent, and temporary colors can be used the same day as any other chemical service.

SPECIAL COLOR PROBLEMS

Brown shades tend to build up on porous ends, while red shades tend to fade easily if ends are porous. This is most commonly explained by the different size of color molecules. To prevent build-up of brown, trim porous ends, color only the new growth during color touch-ups—or remove built-up color from the ends with a mild lightener.

To prevent reds from fading at the ends, use a filler, or, after a retouch, add more red pigment and use a lower volume of peroxide before pulling color through the ends. In a variation on adding red pigment, process the regrowth for twenty minutes, add red with an equal amount of water to the remaining tint and use it on the hair shaft and ends. The water reduces lifting action and allows more red to deposit.

If reds fade quickly along the entire hair shaft, question the client about her lifestyle and the products she uses. Perhaps fadage is the result of sun exposure. When reds fade easily, it is often because the hair is overly porous. Additionally, the ammonia in permanent tints tends to bring out red, orange and yellow in the natural hair—a particular problem with brunettes. The result of overall red fadage is an appearance of brassiness, because when larger red molecules leave the hair, smaller diffused molecules of red, orange and yellow remain and tend to reflect light.

To avoid brassiness in reds, use a lower volume of hydrogen peroxide in your formulation if the desired depth is the same or a deeper level than the natural color. Also, determine if you can achieve the desired result with a semi-permanent color.

To correct a brassy look, you can neutralize it by adding ash tones. Determine if the brassiness is coming from red, orange or yellow and select a shade opposite it on the color wheel. Add a small amount of the neutralizing tint to your shampoo.

If you are adding burgundy tones to dark-colored hair and cannot achieve an intense result, it is because the natural hair is too dark for the formulation you are using. Use a lighter level tint or a greater strength of developer.

REMOVING UNWANTED COLOR

If there is any henna on the hair, it should be removed prior to coloring—particularly if you are using an oxidizing tint. Henna can also interfere with perming and relaxing products, especially if it has been used repeatedly. It should always be removed prior to other chemical services.

To remove henna, use a 70 percent alcohol solution to loosen the henna. Apply it to the hair shaft, avoiding the scalp, wait five minutes, then saturate each strand with mineral oil from scalp to ends. Place a plastic bag over the hair and place the client under a warm dryer for thirty minutes. Next shampoo thoroughly with a build-up removing shampoo, wait three minutes and rinse thoroughly with warm to comfortably hot water. Shampoo again and perform a strand test to determine whether or not any henna remains on the hair.

Metallic hair colors must also be removed from the hair prior to a coloring service. They can be observed by a colored film on the hair shaft or a dull metallic appearance; they can often be felt during a strand test. To test for metallic salts, mix an ounce of 20 volume hydrogen peroxide with a small amount of 20 percent ammonia water and dip a snipping of the hair into the solution. If the hair lightens quickly, appears to begin to melt, has a disagreeable odor or will not lighten at all after thirty minutes, it probably contains metallic salts.

To remove metallic salts, use the procedure that you use to remove henna. You may have to use a heavier oil or a product specifically formulated to remove color—if the hair has not had previous chemical services other than single-process color.

COLOR-REMOVAL PRECAUTIONS

Relaxed and permed hair tends to be porous; therefore, it "grabs" color more quickly, turning darker than desired. While this can be avoided by performing a test strand or formulating color a level or two lighter than the desired final result, colorists commonly end up with too-dark results when coloring relaxed hair. Compounding the problem, some try to correct the error by using a product that was specifically created to remove haircolor, and then recoloring the hair. When the client gets a relaxer touch-up two weeks later, the hair may break off completely, and serious scalp burns could occur.

Color removers are bleaches and should never be used on relaxed hair or hair that has been permed in two steps. Even if hair has been permed with a single-step process, a test strand is essential. Avoid problems in the first place by formulating correctly and performing a test strand; minimize them by using semi- or demi-permanent color on chemically treated hair whenever possible.

COLORING FRAGILE HAIRLINES

Fragile or broken hairlines are common among older clients and those who have a long history of chemical services. Often it is difficult to color these hairlines safely and to apply product to sparse hairlines without tinting the skin. If your client's hairline indicates that a color service would be risky, do not use products that contain ammonia. Test a no-lift product on a hidden area first.

If the client's hairline is sparse or irregular, use an eyelash brush to apply haircolor. With this technique, you can get near-complete coverage without getting color product on the skin.

USING FILLERS

Porous hair acts like a sponge, absorbing liquids faster and reacting to chemicals more quickly. Fillers—from neutrals to bright reds—have molecules that adhere to the hair, filling in spaces in the cortex and helping the color to adhere. Some molecules are also trapped in the cuticle, which helps create an even surface. Fillers even out porosity along the hair shaft and improve the hair's ability to hold color.

Often porosity problems are recognized too late, when color begins to leach out during shampooing. An observant colorist notes the hair's reaction to moisture prior to a color service. Water practically runs off hair that has a very compact cuticle and is not porous. Lack of shine is a tip-off to excessive porosity.

When using red tints, the filler should be applied prior to the service. When performing a double-process blonding service, use a neutral filler to even out porosity. If you've already performed a color service and realize too late that you should have used a filler, try a filler shampoo. To neutralize a shade at the same time, mix the tint that is opposite the undesired shade on the color wheel, a small amount of peroxide, and shampoo, which will dilute the solution. Apply for five minutes and rinse.

Fillers are also used during tint-backs to natural color. If bleached hair might turn green when a brown tint is added (most brown tints are green-based), you can take preventive action by filling the hair with a neutralizing red-orange prior to the application of the brown tint.

DOUBLE PROCESSING

Double-process coloring, during which hair is first lightened to a specific stage and then toned, is most often used to achieve blondes. However, clients who have very dark hair and want a shade that is more than two levels lighter than their natural haircolor generally require double processing. For example, if your level 2 client wants hair that is a true light red, the only way to achieve it without brass and unwanted tones is through a double process.

Clients whose hair is relaxed or curled using a two-step perm should never be given a double-process color.

Whenever double-processing, perform a strand test first and do not lift the hair any more than is necessary to achieve the desired results. Even when using a pale, delicate toner, it is not necessary to pre-lighten hair beyond a level 8.

. . . .

COLORING HAIR THAT HAS BEEN PERMED IN TWO STEPS

Hair that has been permed using a two-step process has been exposed to chemicals twice: once during the straightening process and a second time during the perming process. To color it safely and effectively, Richard Cardone of Richard Cardone Hair Designers and Color Specialists in Pittsburgh, Pennsylvania, uses demi-permanent haircolor.

In this instance, one of the biggest contributing factors to note is porosity. Because the porous hair will have a tendency to grab color and get too dark, offset the problem by formulating with a product that is one or two levels lighter than the desired results. For example, if a natural level 2 client wants a level 4 or 5 gold or red, use a level 7 or 8 product. The results will be high shine with gold tones; it will not be a true level 7 because you are not lifting the hair.

If the client actually wants to change hair color by one or two levels—for instance, from a level 2 to a level 4 warm brown, use a level 6 permanent product with 20 volume peroxide and perform a strand test. If the hair has good tensile strength after the strand test, use this formulation. If you do not like the results of the tensile strength test, perform a second strand test using a level 8 product with 10 volume developer. If the results of this formulation are not satisfactory, stick with safer demi-permanent colors. (Hair that has been permed using a two-step process cannot be lightened by more than two levels, because that would require a double-process color technique, which is incompatible with the perm service.)

To add extra shine and highlights, Cardone uses a "wet-on-wet" technique, in which color is applied over the color, using a foiling technique. When using demi-permanent color, mix a mild lightener with 5 volume developer, weave out sections of hair and apply the formula right over the demi-permanent shade. (Do not use powdered bleaches.) If you are using permanent color, use a level 10 haircolor mixed with 20 volume developer to perform the wet-on-wet technique.

1. To begin, analyze the hair to determine its porosity level; also determine the client's desired results. If a single process will be performed using a permanent haircolor product, perform a strand test first. (Fig. 15.2) If a demi-permanent color will be

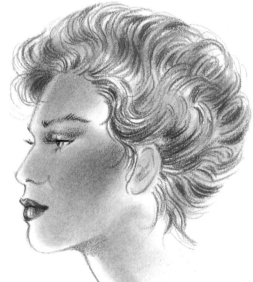

FIGURE 15.1
Before.

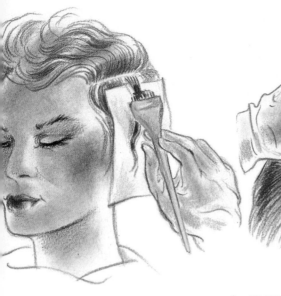

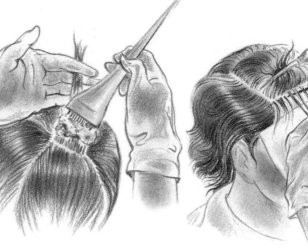

FIGURE 15.2
Perform a strand test. Examine the results.

FIGURE 15.3
Apply the color product to the hair.

FIGURE 15.4
Weave out sections around the face and apply formula directly over previously applied haircolor.

used, formulate the color one or two levels lighter than the desired result.

2. Apply the color product to the hair, using an applicator bottle or a brush-on method. (Fig. 15.3)

3. To add highlights, immediately begin the wet-on-wet technique. When using demi-permanent color, mix a mild lightener with 5 volume developer. When using a permanent color, mix a level 10 haircolor with 20 volume developer. Weave out sections around the face and apply the formula directly over the previously applied haircolor. (Fig. 15.4)

4. Process the base color according to manufacturer's directions. Permanent haircolor usually takes between twenty-five and forty minutes to process. Demi-permanent color takes about fifteen to twenty minutes. Check the hair frequently—particularly if it is porous.

5. When processing is complete, rinse, shampoo and condition. Style using a technique that does not require heat, such as a wet roller set.

TOUCH-UP PROCEDURE

If hair has been permed using a two-step process, you can retouch the curl and the color on the same day if a demi-permanent color product was used. Reperm the outgrowth first. (See Chapter 11 for this technique.) When this process is com-

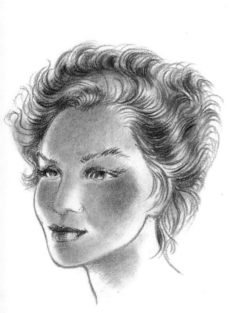

FIGURE 15.5
Finished style, "coloring a two-step perm."

plete, apply the demi-permanent color to the regrowth area only. During the last five minutes of processing, pull the color through the ends to refresh them.

If you used permanent color, avoid same-day retouches. Perform the curl touch-up or recurl first. Wait a week before touching up the regrowth with permanent color.

COLOR PRECAUTIONS FOR RELAXED OR TWO-STEP PERMED HAIR

Whenever coloring hair that has been relaxed or has been permed using a two-step process, keep the following tips from Richard Cardone in mind:

- ◆ Do not try to lighten the hair beyond two levels.
- ◆ Do not use any products that are harsh or abrasive. Use common sense.
- ◆ When using permanent haircolor, use a single-process technique only. Formulate with 10 volume peroxide when staying within the same level; use 20 volume peroxide when changing the color by one or two levels or when covering hair that is over 50 percent gray. Do not use developer strengths above 20 volume.
- ◆ Use fillers if the hair is porous, adding them to your color formula. If the natural haircolor is dark, use neutral-based fillers unless you need to add pigment to the natural hair. (For instance, when it is gray.)
- ◆ Avoid the use of heat during the coloring process; avoid excess heat when styling the hair.

HIGHLIGHTING RELAXED HAIR

It is never recommended that bleach be used on relaxed hair; the hair is often so porous that bleach would lift the color to the orange stage in as little as two minutes. However, you can add face-framing highlights to relaxed hair with a tint. Because relaxed hair is often very porous, causing color to penetrate and grab quickly, apply a protein moisturizer/conditioner to the areas to be highlighted first. This will slow the lightening process, allowing you time to weave out highlights.

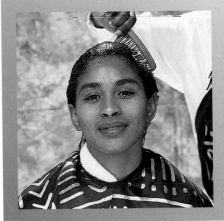

FIGURE 15.6
Comb the moisturizer/conditioner through the hair.

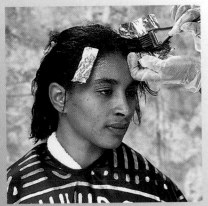

FIGURE 15.7
Weave out the sections around the face and begin application of tint.

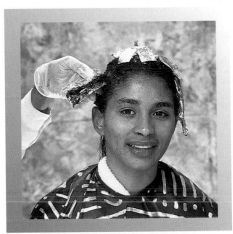

FIGURE 15.8
Check the first foil. Continue to check in five-minute increments.

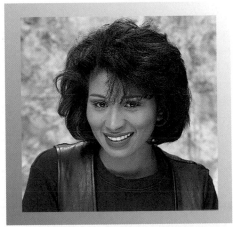

FIGURE 15.9
Finished style, "highlighting relaxed hair."

The following technique from Balmer Galindez, of Salon D 'n' B in New York City, should be performed no sooner than one week after the hair has been relaxed. To be on the safe side, wait two weeks.

1. Shampoo the hair first, towel dry, and, if necessary, place the client under a cool dryer to remove some moisture. When the hair is still damp, part the front section where the hair will be highlighted, redampen the hair if necessary and apply the moisturizer/conditioner by combing it through the hair. (Fig. 15.6)

2. Mix the selected permanent tint with 20 volume peroxide and begin weaving out sections around the face to be foil highlighted. (Fig. 15.7)

3. Work quickly; processing will take from five to fifteen minutes, depending on the hair's porosity.

4. For a natural look, weave out sections to be foil highlighted; for a more dramatic look, slice out sections around the face.

5. After five minutes, check the first foil that you placed. Continue to check this foil in five-minute increments or more frequently, if processing is nearly completed. (Fig. 15.8)

6. When processing is complete, rinse, shampoo and condition the hair; then proceed with styling.

TECHNIQUES FOR MINIMIZING BRASSINESS WHEN TINTING FOR LIGHTER RESULTS

To avoid brassiness when coloring levels 1 through 4 hair, take the underlying pigment into account when formulating. If you use a permanent tint that contains ammonia on virgin hair, the ammonia will cause the underlying pigment to play a greater role in the final result—particularly if you are lightening more than two levels. This is how unwanted warmth gets exposed. (Do not lighten hair that's been relaxed or permed in two steps more than two levels.)

Whenever lightening dark hair more than two levels, Susan Calandro, the color director of Maximus Salon and Day Spa in Merrick, New York, recommends using cool-based colors to mask the underlying red pigment, which becomes more obvious over time. It is the eventual fade-off of these cool tones that causes warmth to become noticeable within a few weeks of the initial service. (To avoid brassiness completely, your best options are to avoid lightening the hair by more than two levels, or, if the hair is in good condition, use a double-process and decolorize the hair prior to toning it.)

Most manufacturers recommend that to predict lift, you multiply the desired level by 2, then subtract the natural level from the result to determine the level tint to use. While this predicts lifting, it does not always result in a cool tone. Therefore, Calandro recommends adding a blue concentrate additive to the formula.

When adding blue concentrates to stave off brassiness, use about a half-ounce of concentrate, but do not add additional developer because of its presence. Follow the manufacturers directions for the developer-to-tint ratio.

If the natural hair is resistant, increase the strength of the developer from 20 to 30 volume and perform a strand test. If the strand test is not satisfactory, increase the strength of the developer to 40 volume for virgin hair, but do not use strengths higher than 40 volume. Keep in mind that the higher volume of developer you use, the more likely it is you will see brassiness; therefore, it is more essential to use a blue concentrate additive and a blue-based tint.

The following technique is for natural level 2 hair, with a desired result of true ash brown. Since the hair closest to the scalp processes faster because of its proximity to body heat, apply the color formula to this hair last.

1. Formulate based on underlying pigment. Use a cool-based color (blue, violet or green) to counteract unwanted warmth. Cool-based colors will appear darker than warm-based colors,

particularly if you are adding a blue concentrate. To account for this, formulate a level lighter than the desired end result.

2. Divide the hair into four sections. Begin applying the color a quarter-inch from the scalp, all the way to the ends. Use a brush-on technique to control the application procedure.

3. Process for twenty minutes or until the hair has reached the midway point of lightening.

4. Remix the formula and apply it to the quarter-inch that was previously left uncolored. Then resaturate the hair shaft and ends. Process until the desired results are achieved; this can take up to forty minutes.

5. Rinse the hair thoroughly and shampoo. If after a week or two brass appears, neutralize it by adding a neutralizing (cool) tint to your shampoo and shampooing the client's hair with it. Also, prescribe an appropriate, cool-based, color-enhancing shampoo and/or conditioner for home use.

MATCHING OR DARKENING NATURAL HAIRCOLOR

If you wish to match the natural haircolor or make it darker, avoiding brass is less difficult than it is when lightening hair, but brassy results are still possible because of fade-off and the action of the developer.

To ensure brass avoidance, apply the previously discussed principles. Select a cool-based tint and add a blue concentrate additive to your formula. When matching or darkening the natural color using a permanent tint, apply the formula to dry hair, using a shampoo-in technique. Process until the desired results are achieved, rinse and shampoo.

COVERING GRAY

About 95 percent of all gray hair is resistant in nature, particularly if the client had coarse hair to begin with. To increase its ability to absorb haircolor, pre-soften resistant gray using an oil bleach lightener with 10 volume peroxide—or 3 percent peroxide to eliminate lightening. For virgin hair with all-over gray, apply the formula to all the hair or to the new growth only if you are performing a color touch-up. If gray is localized, apply the formula to the specific gray areas only. Often even if gray is localized it's safer to apply the formula to all the hair because, while the eye cannot tell, more of the hair is preparing to turn gray and the resistance factor exists. (This is true if the cause of graying is genetic.)

If your gray-haired client wants to cover gray with a light level tint, you may want to use an orange/red filler to pre-pigment the gray after softening it. If during subsequent treatments a larger percentage of the client's hair continues to turn gray, the red may not penetrate as deeply and you'll get an orange effect. Use a deeper red filler on whiter areas, or if you see too much red/orange, use a blue/green color as a neutralizer.

In general, if clients want complete gray coverage, a permanent color is the best solution. Depending on the percentage of gray, its resistance and the desired final effect, semi-permanent colors can be effective, but they can also build up over time, affecting later color results. Semi-permanent gray coverage is best used for male clients, who tend to get frequent haircuts, which removes semi-permanent buildup, and who may have to overcome a fear of peroxide.

Whenever you are covering gray, you are dealing with a "salt and pepper" mix of colors. When using permanent haircolor, you should realize that you will see one result on the pepper-colored hair and another result on the salt-colored hair. Since your results will be dimensional, aim for a pleasing mix.

Francine Castle, who owns Personal Image salon in Wilton, Connecticut, and is a Logics educator, recommends that you look at hair that is 50 percent gray as if you are considering two different heads of hair. If the gray is resistant, she recommends using one of the following three techniques for softening it:

1. Dab on 20 volume peroxide with a cotton ball and wait for twenty minutes. (If the gray is in patches, you can pre-soften the gray only.)

2. Use a gold level 6 permanent color mixed with 20 volume peroxide to pre-soften the hair and impart gold. Apply the formula all over; after about fifteen minutes, towel blot it off and proceed with the color service.

3. Apply the formula you plan to use to color the hair; let it process for fifteen minutes; wipe it off by towel-blotting the hair; and reapply the same formula.

Hair that is 50 percent gray is the most difficult to color correctly, because your decision is not based on whether there is more pigmented hair or more gray hair. If the natural hair is level 3, the primary options are to match the natural color, make it a lighter brown or color it blonde.

Castle says her most common salon request from all women is the blonde option. The first technique that follows is for the client who has relaxed hair; the second is for the client who has had no other chemical services.

GRAY COVERAGE FOR RELAXED HAIR

1. Begin by performing a hair analysis. If the hair is in good condition and shows no evidence of breakage, it can be safely colored using a demi-permanent color product. Demi-permanent colors do not lighten the hair; therefore, the gray hair will take on the color and tone you've selected, and the pigmented hair will be unaffected. (The pigmented hair will not lighten because demi-permanent colors deposit only. It will not darken because the selected color is very light against it—and because there is an extremely slight lightening action from the developer, which is usually undetectable to the eye.) The results will be a blonde highlighted effect.

2. Because relaxed hair is porous and tends to "grab" color, select a color that is two levels lighter than the desired final result. Choose a violet, neutral or gold tone, based on the desired final results and your understanding of the specific product line. Some neutral products will look flat on gray hair; others will not.

3. For hair that is 50 percent gray, mix the demi-permanent color with the corresponding developer, according to manufacturer's directions. (Do not use a permanent haircolor product or it will lift the pigmented hair just enough to give it an orange cast.)

4. Apply the mixture from roots to ends and process according to the manufacturer's directions. Usually, this is from thirty to forty-five minutes. Do not apply heat to relaxed hair or you may compromise its condition.

5. Rinse thoroughly, or shampoo if the manufacturer recommends it; then proceed with conditioning and styling.

GRAY COVERAGE FOR VIRGIN HAIR

1. Level 3 hair that is 50 percent gray can be safely colored with permanent haircolor, if it is has not had previous chemical services. In this blonde-on-blonde technique, a gold-based permanent color is used so that it will slightly lighten the pigmented hair and cover the gray. Then highlights are added throughout the head.

2. To begin, formulate so that the color will lighten the base or natural level from a level 3 to a level 5. To achieve a level 5, some product lines recommend using a level 5 product; others recommend using a level 7 product. Follow the manufactur-

er's guidance for achieving a level 5. Select a violet-based color to control unwanted tones in the gray. Since you are lifting just two levels, you will not get too much unwanted warmth.

3. Mix the color product with 20 volume peroxide and apply it using a virgin application technique. To do this, apply the formula a half-inch from the scalp to the ends and process for twenty minutes. Then remix the same formula and apply it from the root area to the ends. Process an additional thirty-five minutes.

4. Shampoo the hair and towel dry, then select a liquid or powder lightener to use for the highlighting formulation. Mix powder lightener with 20 volume peroxide; mix the liquid lightener with its compatible boosters and developer, according to the manufacturer's directions.

5. Using a foiling technique or a cap, apply the lightening formula to small sections of hair throughout the entire head. For a brightening effect, make the highlights slightly heavier around the face. Check the hair for the desired degree of lightness every ten minutes; aim for yellow to pale yellow.

6. When processing is completed, shampoo, condition and style the hair.

GRAY COVERAGE RETOUCHES

After four to six weeks, depending on how fast the hair grows, your client will need a color touch-up. For hair that has no chemical processes other than color, follow the same steps for the retouch as you did for the initial application. (Retouch the outgrowth only.) If the hair has been relaxed, demi-permanent color can be used the same day as the relaxer touch-up, if the hair is in good condition. If gray requires pre-softening, it is advisable to wait until a week after the relaxer touch-up, to maintain the integrity of the hair.

Same-Day Relaxer and Color Retouch

When performing same-day chemical services, it is imperative that you perform a hair analysis first, to make certain the hair's elasticity and porosity are good. Karen Lafferty, regional training manager for Creative Hairdressers, Inc., in Falls Church, Virginia, recommends that the client avoid shampooing for seventy-two hours prior to a color and relaxer touch-up to minimize scalp sensitivity.

She then selects the strength of relaxer, based on the texture of the hair and the tightness of the curl. The relaxer touch-up is performed first; then a temporary, semi-permanent or demi-permanent color can be safely used to touch-up the color. Because the scalp is sensitive after a relaxer touch-up, towel dry the hair; do not use thermal heat. Coloring the hair when it's damp also helps even out porosity, which is helpful if the hair shaft and ends need refreshing.

1. To begin, part the hair from the center front hairline back to the nape; then part the hair from ear to ear, across the top of the head. Clip the four sections in place. Base the scalp around all four sections, using a light lubricant as a protective barrier. Next move to the crown and take diagonal partings from the crown to the nape, basing the scalp with each parting. Repeat the basing procedure, using diagonal partings that move from the crown to the front hairline.

2. After the entire scalp has been based, apply a protective creme around the entire hairline and the ears. Then apply a reconstructing treatment to the previously relaxed and colored hair shaft and ends to condition them and prevent the relaxing product from overlapping.

3. Take a small amount of relaxer on your glove-covered hand, using it as a palette for the rattail comb. This saves you time during the application. Dip the rattail comb in the relaxer, hold it parallel to your first parting and apply the relaxer. Work from the crown to the nape, taking quarter-inch sections and applying the relaxer to the regrowth. Smooth the relaxer onto the front and back of each section. Work down the center back, then move to the right or left and continue working from crown to nape, using diagonal partings to ensure even relaxation.

4. When the back is complete, work from the crown to the front hairline. Apply the product to the fragile hairline last.

5. When all the regrowth has been covered, begin pressing each section. Using the edge of the rattail comb, take arch-shaped partings from ear to ear and press in an upward motion. Complete the back first; then work from the crown forward.

6. Test the hair at the crown by using the "thumb print" technique. Wipe off the excess relaxer, press your thumb against the hair, toward the head; then lift the hair with the end of the rattail comb and observe the remaining *S*-formation of the curl.

7. When the desired degree of curl reduction has been achieved, rinse the hair with tepid-to-cool water. Use strong water pressure for at least ten minutes. This will combat the product's tendency to adhere to the hair. When rinsing is completed, follow the manufacturer's directions regarding shampoo neutralizing.

8. Towel dry the hair and reapply the constructive treatment along the previously relaxed and colored hair shaft and ends.

Color will be applied to the regrowth only, just as the relaxer was.

9. Use a bowl and brush technique to apply the color. Mix the color product, if you are using semi- or demi-permanent color. (Temporaries require no mixing.) Apply the product to the regrowth, following the same parting pattern that you used for the relaxer.

10. When you reach the nape, take a small section of hair at the back and apply the product along the shaft and ends to determine the degree of color refreshing required. Remember, the reconstructor will slow the process. Continue with touching up the regrowth; after fifteen minutes, wipe the test strand clean and read the color. If the color is even along the shaft and at the ends, fifteen minutes is your correct timing for color refreshing. If the color is not even, adjust your formula according to the amount of deposit desired.

11. If your timing test showed that fifteen minutes of refreshing is required, apply the color to all the hair for the final fifteen minutes of processing. When processing is complete, shampoo the hair and apply a leave-in reconstructive treatment from the scalp to ends. Since the hair has just undergone two chemical services, avoid using thermal heat to style the hair. Use a wet set or a wrapping technique and allow the hair to air dry.

QUICK APPLICATION TECHNIQUES

If it takes two hours to foil highlight a thick head of hair, you minimize your income. The following techniques, from Maureen Clark-Newlove of Noelle the Colour Group in Stamford, Connecticut, process in twenty minutes or less, are perfect for introducing clients to color and work well for a variety of hair types:

SCRUNCH ACCENTS FOR CURLY OR WAVY HAIR

For the dark-haired client, choose a color that is two to three levels lighter than the client's natural hair; for the light-haired client, choose a color that is two to three levels darker than the natural hair. Or choose a color that is the same or one level away from the client's natural color in a different shade or tone. Using your glove-covered hands, scrunch the color into the hair, concentrating on the lower hair shaft. Process twenty minutes and shampoo out. The effect is highlights that occur where color would be naturally diffused by the sun.

BASE BOOSTING

Rather than breaking the base, boost it. Select a permanent color that has the same tonal value as the natural hair but is one level lighter and mix it with 10 volume peroxide. Lather it into the hair, process five minutes and rinse.

AIR BRUSHING

This technique is performed on dry, styled hair. Using a plastic bristle, vent brush and a permanent tint that is one or two levels lighter than the natural haircolor, add highlights quickly and easily. Dip the brush into the color and brush it through the dried and styled hair, following the lines of the client's preferred hairstyle. After twenty minutes, shampoo, rinse and restyle the hair. Highlights will follow the bends and curves of the finished style.

DOUBLE PROCESSING LEVEL 2 OR 3 HAIR

Double processing requires a thorough hair and scalp analysis, and a complete understanding of previous services. Relaxing and perming are incompatible with double processing; previous color services can also adversely affect results. Do not assume that semi-permanent or "temporary" polymer colors will not affect the results of a double process; they will.

Rhonda Hicks, co-owner of Emages by Hair Station U.S.A. in Houston, Texas, and co-founder of the Black Hair Colorists of America, recommends that you perform a double process on virgin hair only. During the consultation, ask your client about all previous services, including henna, to ensure that you are working on a virgin head of hair.

The keys to a successful double process when working with hair that is a natural level 2 or 3 are to work quickly and decolorize only to the stage necessary to achieve your final results. Using a standard first-time application procedure, Hicks leaves a full inch of hair closest to the scalp untouched during the first stage of lightening to allow for product seepage and the fact that the hair closest to the scalp will process very quickly because of its proximity to body heat. As an added safety measure, she uses just one activator or protinator with an oil lightener and 10 volume developer, which allows more control over the procedure than 20 volume does.

The following technique, for level 2 or 3 hair, is for achieving a true level 5 or 6 red with no brassiness.

1. To begin, perform a complete hair analysis as you question your client about any previous chemical services, including

henna and "temporary" colors. If the latter exist, perform a strand test before proceeding with the service.

2. Shampoo the hair to remove any buildup of fixatives or styling aids. Then divide the hair into four equal sections. Even if you are an accomplished colorist, this is essential for control—and because the first section that you lighten may need to be rinsed before you apply the lightener to the final section.

3. Mix oil lightener with one protinator or activator and 10 volume developer. The creamy consistency of the oil lightener will allow greater control during application. Begin applying the lightener at the lower right, back quarter section. (You will proceed in a clockwise manner, from the right back quarter to the left back quarter, and so forth.) Taking very small, one-eighth-inch partings, apply the product from one inch away from the scalp to the ends. If you do not leave a full inch, you risk uneven decolorization, or "hot spots."

4. Work quickly to complete the section; it should take you less than one minute. When the section is completed, wrap a strip of cotton around the perimeter of the entire section to prevent product seepage.

5. Proceed to the next section and repeat the application procedure, taking one-eighth-inch sections. As you work, continuously make a visual check of the first section that you lightened. When it reaches the light brown stage, quickly and thoroughly rinse the lightening product from the hair. Do not lighten to the orange stage or your final results will be brassy and unnatural-looking. (Keep in mind that the tint will lift the hair another level; rinse the hair before you see ANY orange.) Depending on the hair's porosity and the cuticle's resistance, lightening can take anywhere from three to fifteen minutes.

6. To rinse the first section that was lightened without disturbing the second section, use very low water pressure, rinse the hair using a hose attachment and direct the water close to the scalp. Rinse the hair sufficiently to stop the action of the lightener, towel blot it and proceed applying lightener to the other sections.

7. Work clockwise so that your final section will be the top left section. By the time you complete this section, the second section to which you applied lightener may have reached the light brown stage and be ready for rinsing. When the second section reaches the desired stage, rinse it as described in step 6. If the hair is lightening quickly, stay at the shampoo bowl and wait for the remaining two sections to lighten to the desired stage. When the desired degree of lightening has been

achieved, rinse the hair thoroughly to remove the lightening product and towel dry the hair to remove as much moisture as possible.

8. Now apply the lightening product to the hair that is closest to the scalp, which was previously left unlightened. Divide the hair into four sections just as before, and work quickly, applying the product to one-eighth-inch sections. Begin with the right back quarter and work clockwise, continually making a visual check of the previously completed sections. The hair that is within one-inch from the scalp will lighten very quickly.

9. Rinse the sections as they achieve the desired degree of lightness, just as you did during the initial lightener application. Then rerinse all the hair and lightly shampoo it; rinsing alone will not thoroughly remove the lightening product. When you are certain that all the lightener has been removed—particularly at the hairline and around the ears—towel dry the hair and divide it into four sections in preparation for the tint application.

10. To achieve a true red with no brassiness, mix a level 6RG (or 6RO, depending on the product line you're using) with a level 5RV. This avoids too much orange or too much violet in the final result and offsets underlying pigment. Use 20 volume peroxide in your formulation.

11. Apply the permanent tint formula to the hair. Complete each quarter by taking one-eighth-inch partings just as you did before, but this time apply the product from as close to the scalp as you can to the ends. When the application is completed, process thirty minutes, or according to manufacturer's directions. Make a visual check of a test strand frequently when you near the end of the processing time.

12. When processing is completed, rinse the hair thoroughly, condition and style. When working with extremely curly hair, it may be necessary to use a thermal styling technique, such as a press and curl, unless the client wants to wear her hair in a natural. Since you begin with virgin hair and performed an initial hair analysis, the application of heat after a double process should not result in hair damage.

DOUBLE PROCESS RETOUCHING

At least one-eighth- to one-quarter-inch of regrowth is necessary to perform a double-process retouch, so you can avoid overlapping the product onto the previously double-processed hair. To perform a retouch, protect the previously colored hair with a moisturizing conditioner. To decolorize the hair, use a tint bottle to speed the application of the oil lightener; the regrowth is very close to the scalp and will process very quickly. Avoid overlapping product onto the previously colored hair.

Follow the same procedure that you used for the initial application, visually checking the hair frequently. Both the pre-lightening and the tinting processing times will be less than they were during the initial application.

DOUBLE PROCESSING RESISTANT HAIR

When decolorizing hair that has a very compact, glassy cuticle, adjust the timing and the formulation to overcome the hair's resistance. Always perform a strand test first to see if you can achieve the desired degree of lightening.

Test the lightener first, an using oil lightener, 20 volume developer and two activators or protinators. If the cuticle is very compact and the strands are thick in diameter, you may have to process the lightener with heat. Apply the lightening formulation to a strand underneath the hair at the nape, place the client under a medium-warm (never hot) hood dryer and frequently make a visual check of the hair. To achieve a level 5 or 6 result, do not lighten the hair beyond the light brown stage. Check the test strand every five minutes; when you near the desired degree of lightening, continuously watch the hair to avoid over-lightening to the orange stage.

If the lightening process is successful, note the processing time and proceed with the application of the tint to the test strand. Again, make frequent visual checks to determine the correct processing time for the tint. If the test strand shows no contraindications, proceed with the service.

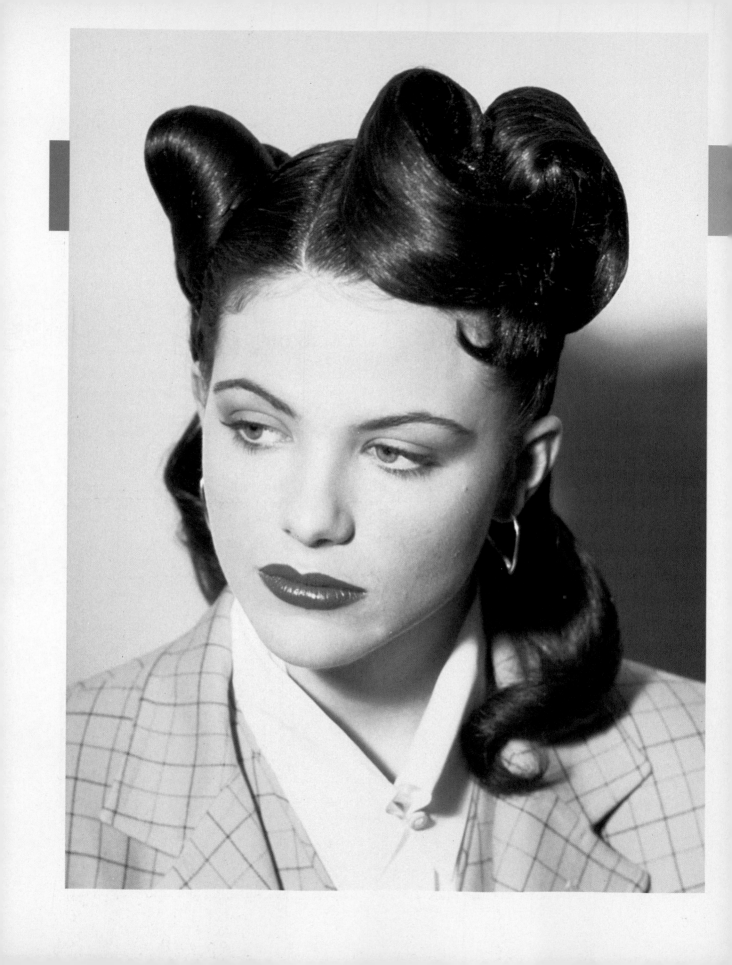

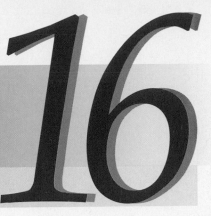

Special Effects Techniques

With hair fiber as your medium, you can craft an astonishing array of highly artistic styles. Classic African hair can be cut into a variety of shapes and quickly shape-changed by selectively picking out or palm-patting certain areas. Any hair type can be wrapped, braided, adorned with ornaments or heavily gelled and sculpted into unique silhouettes.

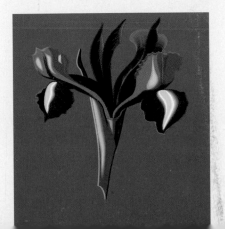

You can also create specialty hairpieces to match your client's own hair—or contrast with it. In creating special styles for your clients, all your artistic skills come into play.

The most likely times that you'll be asked to create a special style are the holidays or when your client has a personal event on the agenda, such as a wedding. If you want to participate in hair competitions, stage shows, fashion photo shoots and other such events, you'll definitely want to develop your special-effects styling techniques.

The following special-effect techniques provide you with a foundation on which you can build your repertoire of skills. Add your own artistic vision, experiment on mannequin heads for fun and a variety of career paths will be open to you.

HAIR WRAPPING

Hair wrapping can be done on long or short hair for a quick accent. It's so popular in the teen market that two entrepreneurs followed the circuit of a nationwide rock tour, paying their way by wrapping hair for five dollars a strand in every city to which the tour took them.

A leather hair wrap or any other narrow strip of fabric can be used to wrap an entire strand of hair, concealing it in the wrap. Younger clients who have long hair frequently like a few sections of wrapped hair sprinkled throughout, for a colorful accent. The technique is simplest on straight hair that is not so fine that it is slippery. If hair has a medium curl pattern, you might want to slick the strand with gel and blow dry it prior to wrapping it.

1. To begin, take a small, square parting. If hair is fine, take a larger section; if hair is dense, take a smaller section. Split the hair into two sections and lay the hair wrap between the two.

2. Cross one section of hair across the wrap; then cross the other section of hair across the wrap in the opposite direction. Then perform a three-strand braiding technique for about half an inch.

3. Now begin to loop the wrap around the remaining hair. Hold the end of the hair tightly between two fingers as you spiral the wrap tightly and evenly around all the hair. Periodically stop looping to gently push the wrap up and adjust it, so there are no gaps that the hair shows through.

4. Continue to the end of the hair and tie the hair wrap at the bottom or use thread to tie the ends and cut off the remaining hair wrap.

NON-CHEMICAL HIGHLIGHTS

Highlights are among the most popular salon services, but some clients are afraid of chemicals; others would love to have highlights just for a night in fashion shades. The solution is to use human or synthetic hair to create effects ranging from micro-lights to chunks of color.

Don Marsella, who co-owns NuWave Salon in the Bronx, New York, and who developed an "Easy Streaks" kit that can be retailed to anyone who wants instant temporary highlights, suggests that the salon service emphasize custom placement and longer-lasting attachment techniques. (His retail kit uses the bonding method.) In the salon, human hair can be custom colored for the client in fashion shades of hot pink, green or blue. For the client who wants a more natural look, the service is ideal when previous chemical services or the hair's condition indicate that chemical highlights would not be advisable.

According to Marsella, the consultation is the most important step to achieve successful results. Establish the client's goals in getting non-chemical highlights, determine the desired effect and describe the choices of hair color and texture. Teens might want one or two strategically placed fashion-shade highlights (in a texture other than their own for a super-dramatic statement); a woman who has relaxed hair might want subtle highlights that will last for weeks.

Next determine how the client will wear her hair to develop a placement strategy. Perhaps she only wants the highlights to show when she wears an updo. Some clients want super-fine micro highlights, while others want a more showy look that will require the use of thicker strands of hair or a denser placement pattern.

The hair's natural texture and curl pattern will guide your choice of attachment techniques. If hair is straight and has a smooth, glassy cuticle, the glue-gun method is your best choice, because this hair won't hold a braid without slippage (unless it is integrated with synthetic fiber). If the hair is naturally curly, the braiding and glue-gun methods work equally well.

The following steps describe what Marsella calls an interlocking method and the glue-gun method. If, after either service, the client thinks more highlights may be desired, you can add them immediately, or if your salon carries the retail kit, suggest the client purchase it and add more highlights at home, at his or her leisure.

INTERLOCKING METHOD

1. After conducting a consultation to determine the client's desires, select human hair in the shade discussed. Divide the

hair into individual strands from super-fine to thick, based on the desired finished effect. (If you're using a weft, cut off the sewn edge prior to dividing the hair.) The techniques for the back of the head and the front of the head vary slightly.

2. Begin at the back, where you will create off-the-scalp braids. Section the hair based on the desired placement. Then part off a half-inch section of hair and divide the hair within it into three separate strands.

3. Take the strand of human hair in the predetermined thickness and position it to join with the right outside strand. (Overlap the ends of the natural hair with the ends of the human-hair addition at least a half-inch.)

4. Smooth the ends and pinch the site of the overlap as you begin a three-strand braid. Cross the right outside strand under the center strand, then continue three-strand braiding a half-inch to one-inch down the strand. Allow the remaining natural and attached hair to fall free.

5. Continue adding highlights in this manner throughout the back, based on the predetermined placement pattern. Then move to the front, where you will create an on-the-scalp braid. Begin at least a half-inch behind the front hairline or the same distance from the natural part line and part a clean quarter-inch-wide section in the desired length. Begin a three-strand, on-the-scalp underbraid. As you work across the curve of the head, pick up natural hair with the outside strand just prior to crossing it under the center strand. After two or three crossovers, add the highlight addition to the outside strands and continue to braid the hair for several more crossovers.

6. Use the above method to add highlights throughout the front until the desired effect is achieved. The highlights can be shampooed along with the natural hair and can be left in for four to six weeks, depending on how quickly the hair grows. If the natural hair is very curly, the highlights may last for eight to twelve weeks because the tight curl takes up much of the new length.

GLUE-GUN METHOD

1. If you have chosen the glue-gun method, begin by shampooing and towel drying the client's hair. Then section the hair, based on the desired design.

2. Part off a half-inch section for the first attachment. Then take a highlight strand in the predetermined

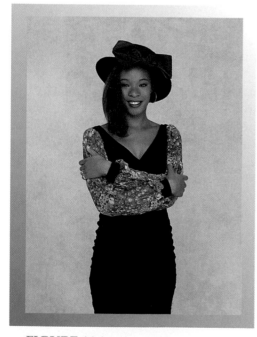

FIGURE 16.1
Special effects hair attached with glue gun.
Photo: Sally Russ for SalonOvations'
Beautiful Black Styles.

thickness. (The service will be much faster if you divide all the commercial hair into individual strands prior to the service.) Cut the ends of the hair to be attached with shears, making certain the ends are blunt. Using the glue gun, apply glue to the blunt ends.

3. Place the highlight strand beneath the small section of natural hair that you parted, positioning it a half-inch away from the scalp. This will help the glue form a smooth, cylindrical bead. Hold the natural hair and the attachment together for a few seconds, until a firm bond is formed.

4. Continue attaching highlights in this manner, based on the pre-planned design. If you used human hair for the highlight attachments, the hair can be styled in any manner desired.

SPECIAL-OCCASION STYLING

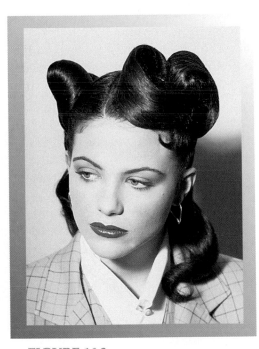

FIGURE 16.2
Creating sophisticated style. Hair: D. Dellaquila for Maximus Salon, Merrick, New York.

When your client has a special event coming up, it's time to use all your artistic skills to deliver a sophisticated style that will stay in place all night. Simple French rolls are the usual option; hairsprays is the tool of choice for making styles long-lasting. But if you want to offer your client something truly unique, consider what makes hair highly malleable. At Maximus Salon in Merrick, New York, D. Dellaquila uses pomade and super-fine hairnets that are practically invisible. These two tools allow you to shape and mold a long-hair design any way you want.

For the style shown here, the hair should be at least seven inches long; ten inches is the ideal length. The look will not work for super-fine hair because some bulk is required in the finished look. However, hair can be of average density, super thick and coarse, or even have slight wave to medium curl. Wavy hair can be blown straight prior to creating the look; an alternative technique for keeping natural wave is also detailed in the following steps.

This 1940s-inspired style is perfect for holidays or proms. If you do not blow dry hair straight first, styling takes approximately forty-five minutes in the salon.

1. To begin, section the hair with an ear-to-ear parting that moves across the top of the head. Allow the back to hang free. Then divide the front into pie-

shaped partings that move from the crown to the front hair-line. You can create as many or as few as you wish, in any size. Part the crown at the back as well, but allow most of the back hair to hang free. For the design shown, the hair is parted on the side; then the light side is divided into one pie-shaped parting, and the opposite side is divided into two pie-shapes. (One is in the front; the other in the back.)

2. Set each section on a large-sized Velcro roller, wrapping it to move down and turn under. Do this when hair is slightly damp, and place the client under a dryer. Then remove the rollers and apply a nickel-sized amount of pomade to the front of the first section. Brush the pomade through the hair, using a brush that combines boar's bristles and plastic bristles for maximum product penetration. Apply another nickel-sized amount of pomade to the back of the section and brush again. Repeat the procedure with all the pie-shaped sections.

3. Separate each section by gathering the hair into elastic bands to create ponytails. Then tie the hairnets to the elastic bands, at the base. Do this by tucking the edge under the elastic band and pulling the net through the loop one time.

4. Now move to the front section of the heavy side. Hold the hair straight up and backcomb the section from the base to the ends, all along the hair shaft. Use a rattail comb to smooth the front surface; then place the hairnet over the entire section and form it into the desired shape, through the net.

5. The net holds the width and prevents the hair from collapsing. You can move the hair within it to conform to any shape by manipulating it with your fingers. For the style show, direct the hair by using your fingers in a circular motion, molding the hair like clay. The pomade allows precise control. Mold the shape and smooth the surface until the desired shape is achieved, then move to the section just behind this one and repeat backcombing and shaping.

6. Complete all the pie-shaped partings in the described manner. Then apply pomade to the top and underside of the back and brush it into the desired shape, allowing the hair to hang free. Curve the ends gently.

WAVY-HAIR VARIATION

If your client has wavy hair, you can use the natural wave to create a Renaissance look, as opposed to one with a 1940s' feeling. Using the same technique, take four partings that move from the front of the crown to the back of the nape. All the hair will be directed back from the front. Roll the ends under to set each section, then proceed as before, combing the hair at the front hairline to lie flat, but maintaining the natural wave. The bands of the ponytails should be positioned at the crown.

CREATIVE DESIGN CUTTING FOR MEN

Extremely curly hair that is cut into the high-top fade, the close fade, the ramp and variations on those styles provides the perfect foundation for special-effects designs. In today's market, even the eyebrows are accented with clipper-cut lines.

For more intricate designs, such as block letters, you should practice on a mannequin head before attempting the design on a person. Clipper control is vital if you intend to create freeform designs. While some companies sell stencils for creating designs, most clients prefer an original.

John Young, a Pensacola, Florida-based educator for the Wahl Corporation, recommends that anyone who wants to cut letters into curly hair take a class, because observation is key. However, to create sharp lines or zig-zags all you need is the right haircut and a steady hand.

The following technique is for enhancing a fade that is between a close fade and a high-top with sharp, Z-shaped lines. To create the basic cut, review the technical instructions in Chapter 7 for the close fade and the high-top fade. In this instance, the front is about one inch high, and the fade is high up the back, almost to the crown.

1. After creating the basic cut, even out the top by freeform cutting from the crown to the front with the clipper blades closed. Then cut a part line in the front center area, not more than a half-inch above the hairline. Slightly more than a quarter-inch is best. Holding the blade in a horizontal position, run it from the area above the mid forehead to the side. Stop when you are just above the front of the ear. The line that is created will be just above the fade line.

2. Go back and redefine the line. Insert the blade into the line, holding the clipper horizontally. If you are right handed, move the blade a quarter-inch to half-inch to the left as you pull it out. (The movement is very slight, but do not pull the blade straight out.) Then move slightly farther to the right and repeat the motion. Move all along the line from front to back, redefining it in this manner. Use short, quick movements.

3. When you have redefined the line two or three times, create the center line of the Z. Position the clipper blade at the end of

the line you just created, angle it down and toward the front and establish the angled line. Do not cut all the way to the hairline—especially if you intend to create a second *Z* within the first one.

4. Redefine this line in the previously described manner. Then position the blade horizontally, at the end of the angled line, and create the bottom line or the base of the Z. Work front to back and establish the line with a single motion as before, then redefine this line, using quick, short strokes.

5. To create a second Z shape within the first one, position the blade horizontally at the center front, about a quarter-inch below the previously cut line. This line will begin almost at the hairline. Create a second Z shape by positioning all three lines an equal distance from the first lines. Cut and redefine them in the same manner as before.

6. You can either leave the ends of the Zs unfinished, so that they end at the side, or continue them toward the back. If you choose the latter option, angle both lines to move back and downward, toward the nape. When you near the nape create smaller Zs that lead off to the very end of the nape.

· ·

WEDDING STYLES

Creating a fabulous wedding style takes more than knowing how to create a classic updo. Today weddings range from first-time, traditional, to second and third times around, casual, avant-garde, theme and historical. Even the word traditional takes on new meaning, as African Americans return to their roots for an Afrocentric "jumping the broom" ceremony, and Asians opt for ceremonies—and headpieces—that reflect their country of origin. Men and women are getting married everywhere from in a chapel to on a roller coaster. As a result, the stylist who creates wedding styles has become a true specialist.

Even if most the weddings in your area are traditional in the Eurocentric sense, specializing in creating bridal styles is one of the best way to get word-of-mouth advertising. Every eye will be on the bride, and her recommendation bears much weight with other brides-to-be.

D. Dellaquila of Maximus Salon in Merrick, New York, has specialized in bridal styling for over ten years. She regularly travels to Europe to learn the latest updos, practices her hair sculpting skills and custom designs headpieces to work with a specific hairstyle.

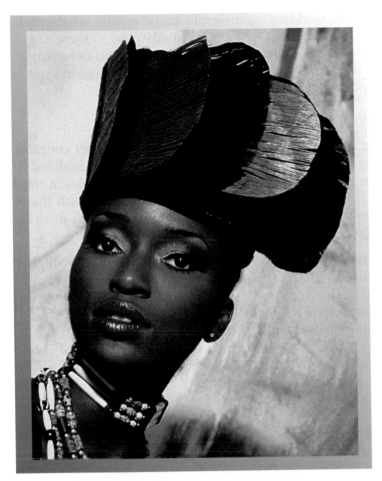

FIGURE 16.3
Fans of hair in multi-colors blend nouveau and native influences.
Hair: Barbara Marshall and Rhonda Hicks for Professional Results
International, Inc. and Emages by Hair Station USA; Makeup:
David Pollard; Photo: George Wong.

She developed the following time line for stylists who work with wedding parties.

PRE-WEDDING TIME LINE

1. Before the bride purchases a headpiece, she should see her stylist to discuss the type of look she has in mind. This is because certain headpieces can only be worn in specific ways. If she purchases a restrictive headpiece and has a particular hairstyle in mind, the two might not go together. For example, a crown is very restricting because it covers the rounds of the head, making it impossible to have a style with full sides. Combs, on the other hand, work with most any style because they can be placed anywhere.

2. Chemical services such as relaxing, double-process coloring and one- or two-step perms should be performed one month before the wedding. This allows curls to relax a bit and avoids disasters, such as a too-curly look, that it's too late to do anything about.

3. Chemical retouches, other than single-process color or a few highlights, should also be performed a month before the ceremony.

4. Three weeks before the wedding, the bride should come in with the headpiece for trial styling. Experiment with different looks if the bride hasn't made a firm decision, and create the style exactly as it will look on the day of the wedding. Also, bridal makeup should be done this day so the bride will see exactly how she'll look.

5. Hair coloring services, other than double processes, should be performed one week before the wedding. There will be no noticeable regrowth, but the hair will have time for porosity to even out. (Artificial nail services should also be done at this time.)

Freeform Curls For Most Any Type of Hairpiece

1. Loose, unstructured curls can be swept up in a freeform fashion to work with almost any headpiece. This style gives a romantic feeling and works best with moderately curly hair. To begin, shampoo and completely dry the hair, then set it on hot rollers. Use medium- to large-sized rollers, and direct all the hair at the front forward. Roll the back lengths under.

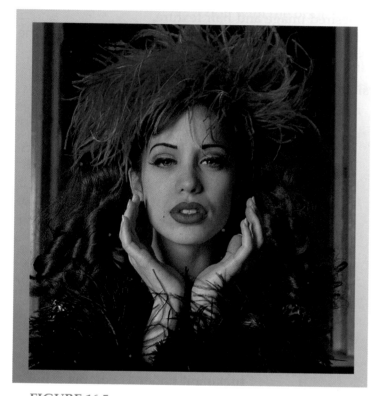

FIGURE 16.5
Spiral curls with a customized hat. Hair: Balmer Galindez for Salon D 'n' B, New York City; Photo: Daria Amato.

2. When the rollers have completely cooled, carefully unwind each roller so the curls remain separate. Liquefy a pomade or cream-base hairdressing between your palms, making sure that you create enough friction to generate heat. (The heat liquefies the pomade and makes it glide through the hair easily.) Then run your fingers through the hair to lightly tousle it. Allow the curls to remain somewhat separated.

3. Next lightly backcomb through all the hair, striving to maintain some curl separation. Mist once with a light hairspray and begin pinning up sections in a freeform fashion. Pick up back sections first; then move to the sides. Determine where to pin up pieces based on the headpiece and the desired final effect. For instance, one back section might be pinned at the occipital and the curls allowed to tumble free; the next back section might be swept up and pinned in place lower on the head.

Classic Option for a Nostalgic Headpiece

1. For a style that has a Grace Kelly feeling, fingerwave the sides and set the back in pin curls. This style is ideal for the woman who will wear a small pill-box hat, a cap or a nostalgic headpiece. The look works well for hair that has some body, is relaxed or is slightly waved. To begin, shampoo and towel dry the hair and distribute gel evenly throughout the head. Determine the placement of the part, which in this case will be

at the side. Begin the first wave at mid-eyebrow level. Position your forefinger at the hairline, just at mid-brow, and comb the first part of the wave upward and back, so a ridge forms against your finger.

2. Next move your finger down about one-and-a-half inches and comb the hair in the opposite direction. Continue placing waves one to one-and-a-half inches apart as you work down the head. Smooth the final wave behind the ear and complete the opposite side in the same manner.

3. Move to the back and comb the hair at the crown down. Planning on three rows of silver-dollar-sized pincurls, determine where your uppermost row should begin. Usually you will begin just above the area where the head curves downward. Part a section wide enough for silver dollar-sized pincurls and comb each pin curl into a *C* shape. The pincurls should rest in the corner of the *C*. When this row is completed, move down to create the second row.

4. Begin at the same side as you did for the previous row, but this time create a backward *C* shape. Again, the pin curls should rest in the corner of the backward *C*. Lastly, complete the final row, using a regular *C* shape. The last row will be somewhat smaller than the previous two.

5. Place the client under the dryer until the hair is completely dry, using a cool setting for the final five minutes. Then remove the bobby pins that held the pin curls and dry mold the hair, following the lines of the set. If desired, apply a light hairdressing, but do not overbrush. Maintain the waves at the sides and the back. Because the hair must hold a molded shape, this design is not recommended for hair that is fine or "pin straight."

WEDDING BRAIDS

With the return of the Afrocentric wedding, braids create an ideal style that stays perfectly in place with minimal fuss. If the client already has braids, they can be designed into a French roll with ease; Goddess and Casama braids, which take about two hours to complete, can be created the day before the wedding.

Laura Little, a stylist and braider at NuWave salon, Bronx, New York, says goddess braids are most popular for several reasons. They are designed to be worn in an updo, which creates a classic wedding style that works with most headpieces. Additionally, since they're large and easy to create, they don't require that an already nervous bride sit for ten to twelve hours to complete a braided style, as she would have to if she wanted numerous small braids. After braids are created, they can be decorated with pearls, roses and colored beads by slipping the decorations onto invisible bobby pins and arranging them around the braids.

If you're unfamiliar with braiding techniques, refer to Chapter 13. After you have reviewed the chapter, use these techniques from Little for creating braided bridal styles.

Goddess Braid Styles

1. To create a goddess braid bridal style, plan for six to eight braids and divide the width of each section accordingly. If hair is fine or lacks density, create eight smaller braids; if it is very thick, plan for six braids. (You don't want the braids to make sparseness obvious.) Begin by parting a wide section that moves from the mid-temple on one side, across the top of the head, to the opposite side. The braids created will swirl around the head.

2. Follow the technique in Chapter 13 for creating the first braid; then base the width of subsequent partings on the total number of braids desired. For each braid, move back and down the head, and follow the lines of the first braid. There should be no large gaps between braids. When you reach the last section, it should move from the left back side to the center of the right side of the head.

3. This style is ideal for a tiara-type headpiece that is worn on the forehead. To decorate it further, slip pearls onto invisible bobby pins and insert them firmly along the braids.

French-Rolled Braids

1. If the client already has numerous free-hanging braids, they can be easily styled into a French Roll. Pull all the braids back, off the face, to the mid-back of the head. Beginning near the top of the section, roll the braids under as a single unit and tuck them under as you secure the roll with bobby pins. Add pearls after the French roll is secured. If desired, let a few braids at the end hang free and curl them under.

2. You can also work from the nape up, but keep in mind that braids can be bulky. Avoid wrapping so that they "stick up" too high on top. View the finished design from all sides. For an alternate version, begin at the top of the head and roll a few braids under. This creates a small "hump" on top. Then create a second roll down the center back.

Quick Braided Design

1. The client who has relaxed or curled hair can have a quick braided design, designed especially for the wedding. This

technique works for any hair type; the only limitation is that it be long enough to pull back into a ponytail. To begin, comb all the hair straight back and secure it into a high ponytail.

2. Take pre-braided sections, wrap them around the base of the tail and secure them; then spiral the braids around the pony-tail, completely covering it. Roll any free ends under and clip them up if desired. Use enough braids to cover the ponytail, so you get a thick cone effect. The style will support decorative pearls or fresh flowers; it also works well with a crown-type headpiece or tiara. Netting can be attached at the base of the ponytail.

CREATING YOUR OWN HAIRPIECES AND ORNAMENTS

Custom hairpieces and hair ornaments are easy to create, if you have a hair weft, water-soluble glue and a free countertop. Custom pieces allow you to create the ultimate special-effects styles, because no one will create an ornament or hairpiece exactly like you do. It's also a great way to make use of excess hair from pre-ordered wefts. If you have a long four-inch-wide piece of a weft left over, turn it into a custom-shaped ponytail.

Hairpieces can be created with strong-hold gel, which allows you to gently comb through them; ornaments can be cut into any shape if you apply glue to weft prior to cutting out the shapes.

What follows are the basic techniques for creating an out-of-the-ordinary ornament and a custom-shaped hairpiece from a human hair weft. Some synthetic hair may also work well.

HUMAN-HAIR ORNAMENTS

1. Place a hair weft on top of aluminum foil on a flat counter top and carefully comb it from the ends up to the sewn edge to smooth the hair and remove tangles. If necessary, spritz lightly with water from a spray bottle and recomb two or three times.

2. Next use a wide brush for applying haircolor and brush water-soluble glue evenly onto the entire weft. Work from the sewn edge to the ends, moving from one side to the opposite. Make certain the glue is evenly distributed and that all the hair is covered.

3. Lay a second piece of foil over the top of the hairpiece and carefully flip it over in one smooth motion. (Hold the edges of

the foil and the sewn edges of the weft together, taking care not to bend the ends of the hair. You can also flip the piece without placing a second piece of foil on top; be sure the piece of foil under the weft is large enough that it does not pull up with the hairpiece.) Quickly smooth the opposite side with the back of a comb and apply glue to it.

4. Slip a heat concentrator attachment on your blow dryer, set it on medium heat and use it to dry the glue. When the first side has dried, carefully lift the hairpiece, place it on a clean piece of foil and dry the opposite side.

5. The hair should be stiff enough to cut shapes from, but the color of the weft will be evident once the glue has dried. You can now cut out any shape desired to create an ornament.

6. For a flower, use a pre-cut cardboard petal as your pattern. Cut out several human hair petals and glue them one-by-one to a stem that can be inserted above a chignon or pinned into the hair. Or cut out a large teardrop shape and "fluke" it by using a curling iron to curve the edges inward. With a little imagination, you can create butterflies or various other shapes that can then be decorated with glitter, beads, mini gems and other items.

CUSTOM HAIRPIECES

1. A weft of any length or width can be molded over a specific shape to create a short or long hairpiece. If you have a long weft that's about four-inches wide, comb it to remove any tangles. Then apply a strong-hold gel, combing it through evenly from sewn edge to ends. Don't apply so much gel that you get flaking; use only as much as you'd use on real hair.

2. Insert a ball or a lightbulb under the weft, closest to the sewn edge. Tie the hair tightly at the sewn edge or secure it with a rubber band. Push the ball or bulb as close to the band as you can get, comb the hair evenly over it and position another rubber band near the base of the rounded part of the bulb or at the end of the ball.

3. Insert a second, smaller bulb or ball as close to this rubber band as you can, underneath the weft. (Bulbs should stack up on one another with the rounded portion nestled in the stem of the previous bulb.) Continue the procedure as you work down the hairpiece, using progressively smaller bulbs or balls. (You can use same-sized bulbs or balls if you're good at balancing them close to one anther.) Apply a small amount of extra gel at the ends, and shape the ends into a gentle curve. Allow the gel to dry naturally or speed dry by using a blow dryer and your concentrator attachment.

CHAPTER 16 SPECIAL EFFECTS TECHNIQUES ◆ 255

4. When the gel is completely dry, carefully remove all the bulbs or balls and lightly comb through the rounded shapes so they don't appear stiff. Mist the entire piece with finishing spray, a hair shiner or lacquer for extra hold. The hairpiece can be attached by inserting bobby pins through the bands closest to the sewn edge. Conceal this site with natural hair.

CHEMICAL SERVICE ADJUSTMENTS FOR THINNING HAIR

If hair is thinning noticeably and the client desires chemical services, take extra precautions. Always perform a strand test to predict outcome and a patch test to determine allergic reactions.

When perming thinning hair, use zig-zag parting patterns to avoid the separation between rods that can reveal the scalp. If you roller set or iron curl the hair after perming, use zig-zag partings with these tools as well. A client who is losing hair and wants a perm should be taught to style it by using moisturizing styling creams. These products prevent hair from drying and avoid the lines of demarcation that rollers can produce.

If the client wants to continue relaxing the hair, leave some of the wave pattern in the hair. If you were previously relaxing the hair to 90 percent, try reducing the curl pattern by 80 percent When perming the hair in two steps, use larger rods and zig-zag partings, and always perform a strand test.

Haircolor can actually benefit thinning hair; henna rinses or demi-permanent color gently create the illusion of thicker strands. In general, avoid overuse of chemicals and heavy gels, which can build up or make combing more difficult. The less tugging or pulling on thinning hair, the better.

While scalp massages may increase the blood circulation and nourishment to the hair shaft, there is no evidence that these types of treatments prevent hair loss or cause hair that has stopped growing to start again. If balding is hereditary, they are of no use. However, if stress is causing hair loss, a relaxing scalp massage can't hurt.

CAMOUFLAGE CUTS

One of the simplest ways you can use your skills to assist the hair-loss client is to create a cut that camouflages thinning hair. In general, shorter cuts give thinning hair the illusion of thickness.

Often men's hairlines recede in a horseshoe shape. As a result, the bulky center section draws attention to the receding areas on either side. If you soften this weight line and cut the hair into a close, squared shape, the receding areas appear more balanced.

Daniel Ruidant, who co-owns Le Hairdesign College in Dallas, Texas, and who has specialized in hair replacement techniques for over twenty years, adds these tips for creating camouflage cuts, either alone or in conjunction with chemical services:

◆ For hair loss at the crown, cut the sides and nape very close. This creates the illusion of a fuller top.
◆ Taper and texturize straight hair with a razor or thinning shears; if the hair is curly, use thinning shears.
◆ When using thinning shears, use an average-sized shear with about forty-two teeth; don't use channel shears. Always hold the section and the shears vertically; if you cut horizontal sections, you'll get undesirable lines in the cut.
◆ For a receding front hairline, avoid the low side part and "comb-over" approach. Remove any bulk in the center and cut the hair, following the natural growth patterns. Style the hair for fullness, not so it moves straight back.
◆ For men or women, this is a great time to introduce a soft perm for added fullness. Use zig-zag partings and alternate the directions of the wrap. Direct the first row forward, direct the second row back, and so forth. Select the rod size based on the hair's texture.
◆ For men who have fine or thinning hair, the ideal length on top is two to two-and-a-half inches.
◆ Male pattern baldness follows specific patterns; women tend to get a diffused effect with hair loss because the hair loss pattern is the same throughout the entire head. For women who are losing hair, the ideal length is no more than three-inches. The sides and nape should be close and tapered to emphasize fullness on top, which a perm can enhance.
◆ If the hair is super curly, texturize it to 50 percent. Depending on the natural growth pattern, loosened curl may conceal some of the hair loss.
◆ When hair loss has reached 50 to 75 percent, a hair integration system is ideal. The curlier the hair, the easier it is to blend the natural hair with the integration piece. (The same is true of hairpieces.)

The following steps provide a general guideline for creating a men's camouflage cut for a receding hairline. Adjust the technique by hair type and the degree to which the hairline is receding. Always work with natural growth patterns.

MEN'S CUT FOR A RECEDING HAIRLINE

1. If the hair is straight, do the entire cut with a razor, which will add lift and movement. First cut the sides horizontally, as you very slightly project the hair. Use a slightly diagonal forward line and cut the hair to just above ear length. (If hair is very curly, use thinning shears and a vertical parting pattern.)

Establish the guide, then cut uniform lengths up to the receding area. Cut the entire side up to the receding area if you are using vertical partings. Repeat the procedure on the opposite side.

2. At the receding area, part a small hairline section to remain free. Then blend the receding area to the sides by slide cutting. Move in the direction the hair naturally grows, and do not cut it too short. Repeat blending on the opposite side. This maintains length in the receding areas.

3. Next part the lower back and cut the hair close, continuing to use the razor for straight hair. Cut a short, close nape line; then cut the hair above it, using fine partings. If the hair is wavy or curly, you may want to use vertical or angled partings for a better blend.

4. When you near the occipital, angle your fingers to create a length increase and continue cutting, working toward the top of the head. When you reach the top, trim the ends if necessary. The hair in front should increase in length as it moves back toward the crown.

5. Now blend the hair between the shortest and longest points. Make certain the hair is well blended behind the ear and above it, so that it does not stick out at the ears.

6. Recheck the front to make certain the center fringe is not too long or bulky—particularly if the receding area creates a strong horseshoe shape. Use curved partings in front and cut from one receding area to the other, using low projection.

7. Reduce bulk in the center and blend the hair to the receding areas. To conceal receding areas even more, part the hair on the side and taper the hair to move toward the opposite side. If the hair is curly, do not razor taper. Instead, cut the hair so there is no bulk in front and explore chemical texturizing options with the client. When the hair is texturized, the curl will elongate and may help camouflage receding areas.

CREATING CUSTOM HAIRPIECES

When large areas of the scalp become bald or extremely fine (sometimes the hair produced is little more than fuzz), a camouflage cut is no longer an option. Frequently, men turn to the extreme comb-over, because no one has suggested a better option—the hairpiece. The approach to creating custom hairpieces varies from manufacturer to manufacturer, as do attachment techniques for hairpieces. If you wish to create hairpieces for your clients, it is always recommended that you take a class, since nothing replaces hands-on experience. However, if you'd like to assess your interest and skill in this area, the following steps, from Daniel Ruidant, demonstrate what is required to create a custom hairpiece.

1. The size and shape of the balding area is most important. To document it for a hairpiece manufacturer, place plastic wrap over the client's head and trace the outline of the area that the headpiece will cover. Do not trace the precise lines; overlap the sides with the actual hair so the tracing is a bit larger than the actual balding area. An alternate technique is to create a plaster of Paris mold of the area.

2. Send the tracing or mold to the manufacturer, along with a sample of the client's hair. Include notes on specific growth patterns, directions, texture, color and density. The hair sample should large enough to be representative so that the manufacturer can match it. If hair differs widely between the nape and crown, take two samples and note from where each sample was taken. Alsonote the desired curl pattern. The client may want a perm and a hairpiece to match it; curly hair blends better with hairpieces.

3. Prior to ordering, discuss types of bases and attachment methods with your client. The best choice of base for the active client who exercises, participates in sports or perspires easily is a thin, ventilated base. These bases are more delicate but are also more natural looking. "Breathable skin" bases are extremely light, soft and natural. If the client has a medical condition, a hard base will protect the scalp better. The most common form of attachment is double-stick tape; the more active client may prefer spring clips or a weaving attachment, if enough natural hair is left. Also discuss the chosen fiber with your client. Hairpieces that are made of synthetic hair are less expensive, and some of the newest synthetic fibers can be heat styled and will accept up to 360 degrees of heat. When ordered in a specific curl configuration and texture, synthetic pieces are easiest for the client who has minimal styling dexterity. (Always order synthetic hair for clients who have very curly hair or you'll have to continually reperm the hairpiece.) Human hair pieces can be permed, colored or thermally styled, but can lose their color if the client lives in a geographic area that has lots of sunshine. They must be regularly reserviced if they are chemically altered.

4. For straight hair, the longest-lasting and strongest attachment technique involves bonding. The bonding technique is performed in the same manner in which hair wefts are bonded to

the hair. (Refer to Chapter 12.) Cut the hair around the perimeter of the hairpiece to one-eighth-inch, apply the bond directly to the hair and the perimeter of the hairpiece and seal the two together. When the hair grows out, remove the bonding, clean the hair and the hairpiece, recut the hair and rebond the hairpiece. This attachment technique lasts for four to six weeks.

5. Curly hair can be integrated with the hairpiece through a weaving technique. Let the manufacturer know that you want the hairpiece to be manufactured with nylon loops around the perimeter. (The company may ask for specifications on size.) When the hairpiece arrives, braid the natural hair through the loops, using an integration technique. Pass the hair through the loops as you braid a track all round the hairpiece. This technique cannot be used with straight hair, which tends to slip out of the braids. For curly hair, the technique lasts as long as two months.

6. When the hairpiece arrives, double check the measurements, color, density and curl configuration. If the hairpiece meets all the standards to which it was ordered set up an appointment for the fitting and conduct it in a private area of the salon. After checking the fit on the client, cut the hairpiece as desired. Keep in mind that a real hairline is very light. Do not cut a heavy box shape or the hairpiece will not look natural.

7. Razor cutting the front hairline will help make it appear more natural. Do not use a razor on synthetic fibers, or you'll get frizzy-looking results. Cut the hairpiece longer than you want it to be in the final cut, so that you can more easily avoid errors. (If you cut it too short, the piece is ruined.) Most men prefer a hairpiece that is no longer than three-inches on top, which is then cut to two or two-and-a-half inches. Blend the hairpiece to the natural hair, texturize the sides and back, then retrim the shape, if the client desires.

8. Advise your client on home care of the hairpiece. Synthetic pieces should be washed in cold or tepid water and shampooed with a product that is especially formulated for synthetic hairpieces. After thorough rinsing, synthetic hairpieces should be towel-blotted and placed on a wig stand to dry. They should never be brushed when wet if they were created to match natural curl. (The curl will relax.) Recommend professional shampoos and conditioners for human hairpieces and instruct your client to lightly towel blot it and allow it to dry on a wig stand.

9. Reschedule an appointment for the following week so that you can make certain your client is happy and you can check

the hairpiece to make certain the client is cleaning it correctly. Every six months, hairpieces should be sent to a professional for cleaning and reconditioning. Special ovens are used for this, and most manufacturers can recommend a professional hairpiece cleaner.

HAIR-LOSS SOLUTIONS FOR WOMEN

Women who have thinning hair have many of the same options as men. Cuts that conceal the thinning area, body perms and creative styling techniques all come into play. Younger women often favor hair integration systems. (They work for men, too.) These light pieces have an open mesh base and look somewhat like hairnets with large open areas. Integration systems, which come pre-made— or can be custom ordered or handmade—have hair attached to the base. The client's natural hair is pulled through the venting and is integrated with the hair from the integration piece. They're excellent for a woman who has allover thinning and can also be designed for clients who have specific-pattern balding. Since integration systems can be created with bangs and cut so the hair falls forward, they're also ideal for the client who has a fragile hairline or even severe hair-line breakage. The hairline is concealed and allowed to restore itself, if damage is not permanent.

HAIR INTEGRATION SYSTEMS

Custom integration systems have webbing that is usually crocheted. Hair of any length, texture, curl configuration or density can be added along the lines of the base or webbing. This allows you to add more hair wherever it is needed and even make adjustments for changes in texture within a single head of hair.

Lois Christie of Christie & Co. in Bayside, New York, specializes in custom-made integration systems. According to her, systems can be created for any hair type. Hair knows no nationality; under-standing the varieties of hair texture is essential for creating custom integration systems. Even a client who has 75 percent hair loss can wear an integration system; only large bald areas are a contraindi-cation for using one.

Christie recommends taking at least an hour for the consultation to discuss cost, the procedure, realistic expectations and mainte-nance. Systems average between 750 and 1,500 dollars and general-ly must be replaced twice a year.

Once the client understands the system, a mold is created, just as it is for a hairpiece. Secure plastic wrap over the head with a band

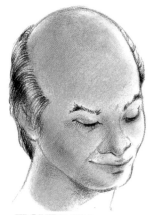

FIGURE 17.1
Before.

and mark the areas of hair loss with clear tape and marker, noting where the perimeter of the base will end, where more density is desired and so forth. This mold is sent to the manufacturer along with a sample of the client's hair and notes on its texture, color, curl configuration and percentage of gray. A mesh base with a blend of synthetic and human hair is created.

According to Christie, it is best to apprentice at a salon or take classes where available, so that you understand venting, molding, working with all types of hair texture and working with the hairpiece. While suppliers can make adjustments or sell you pre-made pieces, it's ideal to perform final custom fitting in the salon.

Attachment methods for integration systems are similar to those available for hairpieces. They can be sewn onto tracks, as long as the client has enough natural hair to create the tracks, or they can be bonded to the natural hair. This method lasts four to six weeks. They can also be attached with spring clips or locking combs if the client wishes to remove the piece at night.

When the system arrives, it generally has more hair than desired so you can cut and taper it. It's rare you'll want to add more hair, if you provided detailed instructions on density for the manufacturer. The following steps detail the procedure after the custom-made piece has been ordered and include Christie's tips for working with integration systems.

1. Perm, color or relax the client's remaining hair before the system arrives. Any wave or curl helps the system blend better with the natural hair, although it can be straight. If the client wants relaxed hair and a system to match, leave some body and movement in the hair; don't relax it bone straight. It's best to perform chemical services before ordering so the piece precisely matches the client's hair.

2. When the integration system arrives, place it over the client's head and check the fitting, based on the attachment technique that will be used. It may take two to three fittings for the piece to fit perfectly on the head. Also make certain the piece was created to all the specifications ordered, in terms of color, density and curl configuration. Pull the client's hair through the piece to check your blend.

3. If the client has enough remaining hair, create a track to which the system will be sewn. The track should be a half-inch to one-inch behind the front hairline, depending on the hairline's density. Begin at the front and create an oval or *U*-shaped track all round the head. If the hair is fine or weak, incorporate synthetic fiber into the track to strengthen it, using an interlocking technique. For a better, stronger fit, begin at the

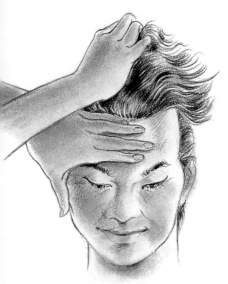

FIGURE 17.2
Press system to natural hair.

crown and create circular tracks. Plan for three to four tracks that end about an inch from the hairline, where the integration system will end. Follow the same pattern for bonding, placing adhesive on the natural hair and the perimeter of the system.

4. If you created tracks, sew the system onto the tracks, using thread in a color that matches the client's hair. If the system is bonded to the hair, press the system to the hair until the bonding sets, then allow it to dry. (Fig. 17.2) If you are using a temporary attachment technique, show the client how it is done. After attaching the piece, pull the hair through the webbing and distribute it evenly.

5. Next proceed with cutting. Take partings with great care and cut the system with the client's hair. Cut it a bit longer than desired at first to avoid costly mistakes. Taper the hairline to remove bulk and create a natural-looking blend. If the piece combines human and synthetic hair, which is the most natural-looking mix, do not use a razor. (Since chemical services fade on human hair, the system will "fade" with it and appear more natural as time goes by.) Hair with some wave and/or layering conceals the mesh base best; avant-garde cuts, such as highly asymmetric cuts, should be avoided. Clients will be happiest with a cut that allows styling versatility.

6. Style the hair as desired, avoiding tension. Do not stretch the hair when it is wet. Today's synthetics can withstand heat styling, but take care not to over-concentrate heat in one area. As you work, show the client how to style the hair and how to lightly comb it without pulling on the system. Pay particular attention to avoiding pulling at the hairline.

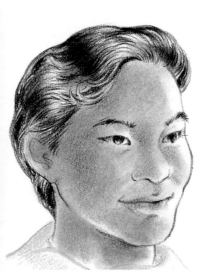

FIGURE 17.3
After: hair integration is complete.

7. Discuss home care with the client. Christie relates care of the system to care of your finest silk blouse. Gentle shampooing should be performed with a mild cleanser. Overuse of conditioners should be avoided or slippage might occur. Instruct the client to condition the ends of her hair only and avoid oil or lanolin-based conditioners. Application of light gels and minimal use of hairspray will extend the life of the system; mousses tend to get gummy on the synthetic hair. Clients who have relaxed hair should avoid overuse of oil-based products and styling creams, since these could also cause slippage in the tracking. The system should be adjusted in the salon every four to six weeks, depending on the rate of hair growth. At that time, chemical touch-ups can be performed. No matter how delicately the hair is handled, it will not last a lifetime; the client should plan on ordering a new system twice a year.

HAIR ADDITIONS FOR SPECIFIC HAIR-LOSS PATTERNS

Hair additions provide another excellent option for women. Wefts can be added where they're needed; even if there is a completely bald patch on the head, the thread weaving technique can be used to extend the track across an area where there is no hair.

The following placement pattern is for adding hair additions for the woman who has a thinning patch at the crown. It can be adapted for men, using wefts that are cut short and selected match the client's natural texture. (If you require more detailed braiding information, refer to Chapter 13.)

Techniques for Hair That Is Thinning at the Crown

1. Perform a hair analysis to make certain there is sufficient healthy hair surrounding the thinning area to safely create a braided track. Examine the condition of the scalp and its flexibility and make certain there is no hair breakage.

2. Select a weft of synthetic hair that matches the client's natural color, texture and curl configuration. Part about an inch of the client's front hairline. Then create an oval-shaped part that moves all around the thinning area. There should be at least a half-inch of hair inside the oval part. Work toward the back, around it and up the opposite side, striving for a uniform shape.

3. You can either create a braid that follows the circular pattern, using the standard tracking technique, or incorporate a very fine section of synthetic hair into the braid, if needed. To do the latter, take a long section of synthetic hair, fold it in half and position the *U*-shape just above the first piece of hair to be braided. Take the synthetic hair along with a strand that will be the outside strand of the braid and cross the two under the center strand, together. Do the same with the opposite side of the synthetic strand and the section of hair that will be the other outside strand.

4. Continue braiding, using an underbraiding technique and following the curved parting. Each time you pick up a new outside section for the braid, incorporate it with the synthetic strand.

5. The braid should be no wider than a half-inch. Work toward the front, then around the opposite side to the back. When the two ends meet, tie and snip off the synthetic strand and reinforce the junction site by stitching the two together. Run the thread through the knot at the end of the synthetic hair for a smooth junction and keep the site as flat as possible. Reinforce

the braid and keep it flatter to the head by continuing to sew all around the braid, using a slip stitch.

6. Add a second circular braid if desired, but do not go any closer than a half-inch from the front hairline. Then take a pre-measured weft of hair (allowing an extra half-inch for error) and sew it to the first track. Review Chapter 12 if you are not familiar with sewing wefts onto tracks.

7. Clip this hair up out of the way and sew the second, longer weft to the outer track, if you chose to create two. Now gently comb all the hair back and cut the hair as desired.

HAIR ADDITIONS FOR HAIR THAT IS THINNING ALL OVER

If the client's natural hair has thinned all over and the hairline has begun to recede, all the remaining hair on the head can be incorporated into braids, to which wefts will be attached. In this technique, very wide partings are used to incorporate enough hair to create a braid. (The width depends on how thin the hair is.) The technique is not recommended if there is hairline breakage. It is ideal for fine or mature hair, but may not be the best solution if actual bald patches exist.

Each parting will be about a quarter-inch to a half-inch wide, depending on how much hair you have to work with. Braids are created around the entire circumference of the head, working from the hairline to the crown in progressively smaller circles. Then wefts are attached. A layered cut that includes bangs conceals all the tracks. Human hair wefts may work best with this technique, because the layers can easily be iron curled or blow dried for added volume.

1. To begin, perform the hair analysis. If there are no contraindications, begin braiding about an inch above the nape. Since thinning hair often has an irregular hairline, adjust how far up you move so that fragile hairs are left free. Smooth the hair above this section and clip it up if necessary to keep it out of the way.

2. Work around the entire head, creating a small, smooth under-braid. When you have braided the hair all around the head, tack down the hair where the two ends meet. Tuck any strays underneath the braid and use a slip stitch to sew around them.

3. Now create the next braid about a half-inch above the first one. All the circular braids should be the same distance apart; make adjustments based on how much hair is on the head. Keep in mind that all the hair will eventually be incorporated into small, smooth braids. (The braids themselves are no more than a quarter-inch.)

WIGS FOR TOTAL COVERAGE

Often mature clients, those who have a form of alopecia or clients undergoing chemotherapy prefer full wigs to hairpieces. Once salons dominated the wig business; today boutiques, department stores and mail-order houses have taken most of the business. However, these firms cannot cut and style the wigs, nor can they prescribe a proper program for wig care.

Salons that choose to sell wigs should carry a large stock of diverse colors, styles and hair types. Even if you don't retail wigs, you'll often be asked to cut or style them. Wigs can be synthetic or human hair, and the cutting and styling techniques for each vary.

CUTTING WIGS

Prior to cutting any wig, section the hair and wrap it into flat pin curls before placing the wig on the client. This reduces bulk. If the client has super curly hair, you may want to blow it straight first.

The simplest parting pattern is to separate the back from the front with an ear-to-ear parting and divide the front into three sections of equal size. Then divide the back in half, horizontally, and pin all the sections into flat pin curls. Next place the wig on the client's head and make certain it won't slip.

If the wig was custom made to match the client's hair, chances are you'll have very little cutting to do. If the wig was pre-designed it may require more cutting, because these wigs often have excess bulk at the crown, which you'll need to lighten.

Human hair wigs can be cut much like the client's hair, only you must be watchful for slippage. Account for this by taking small sections and continuously checking the position of the wig. Synthetic hair takes some getting used to. Synthetic wigs are usually pre-styled and the hair tends to stay in the pre-designed position, so there is rarely a need to clip it out of the way. Do not use razors on synthetic hair because it will frizz unnaturally. Tailor the perimeter first; then lighten the interior.

WIG CARE

Wigs should be washed as often as a client washes her own hair. Human hair wigs can be shampooed and conditioned, colored, permed and cut just like your client's hair. If your client wants to style the wig at home, show her how to secure it to a wig stand and blow dry or iron curl it. These wigs can be lightly shampooed in a basin, conditioned, thoroughly rinsed, towel-blotted and lightly combed before they are placed on the stand to dry.

Synthetic wigs should be washed only with shampoos that are specifically formulated for synthetic wigs. First gently brush the wig to dislodge any large particles. Synthetic wig fiber will spring back to its original shape, so don't worry about disturbing curl. Next pour a small amount of the shampoo into cool water, turn the wig inside out and dip it in and out of the water several times before allowing it to soak. After about five minutes, rinse the wig thoroughly under cool water as you gently squeeze out suds. Then blot the wig carefully with a towel.

At this point the wig should still be inside out. Turn it so that the right side is out, gently shake it and place it on the wig stand. Do not brush or comb synthetic wigs when they are wet. When the wig is completely dry, it can be lightly brushed until the style springs back. If you apply heat to synthetic wigs, make certain the fiber is one of the modern ones that can withstand heat.

According to Audits and Surveys, a New-York-based research firm, total retail sales in salons stands at 2.7 billion dollars—a fraction of total sales. (Consumers spend more than half that amount on shampoos alone at non-salon outlets.)

Many salons have consistently failed to retail in large numbers because of inadequate education in prescribing product. Owners, who are most often working stylists, have minimal business training in retailing, product display, merchandising and promotion. Stylists rarely receive education in the importance of prescribing products and often consider themselves artists whose image would be tarnished by selling products.

But savvy stylists can significantly increase their incomes by retailing, and today's sophisticated salons use retail sales to fund employee benefits packages.

For those who have never learned to retail properly, the picture just got worse. That's because, with the changing composition of the population, salons that barely grasp elementary retailing concepts will have even more to learn about prescriptive retailing to the market segments that are growing the fastest.

However, if you understand different hair types, the effects of all chemical services and the principles of prescriptive selling, you'll be prepared to succeed in all professional areas as the market evolves.

ANALYSIS-BASED, PRESCRIPTIVE RETAILING

Take-home retail products are your service insurance. If your client has received a perm, color or relaxing service but was not prescribed the correct products to properly maintain what's been done to the hair, faded color, prematurely relaxed perms and dried or damaged hair could result. Clients who wear braided styles need special braid oils and scalp moisturizers, and they are going to buy them somewhere. It is best if they buy from you and receive proper instruction in their use.

Prescribing products based on hair analysis requires product knowledge (including an understanding of product ingredients) and a complete understanding of the client's needs. Those needs are not only based on hair type and condition but on the client's personal preference, lifestyle, home styling ability and desire to receive professional recommendations. In several surveys, consumers indicated that they would try a product if their professional stylist recommended it.

After a client has received a service in your salon, check your notes on the client record card. The record card should include information on:

◆ The hair's texture. Is it fine, medium or coarse? Is the texture at the hairline different than the rest of the strand, or the same?
◆ Density. Is the hair sparse or thick and abundant?
◆ Porosity. Is the hair resistant, average or overly porous?
◆ Tensile strength or elasticity. How much will the hair stretch before the strand breaks when the hair is wet? When it's dry?
◆ Overall type. Is the hair dry, normal or oily? What about the scalp and the ends? Just as you can have dry skin with an oily T-zone, you can have an oily scalp and dried ends.
◆ Overall condition. Is the hair healthy or damaged?
◆ Previous services. Is the hair virgin or is it chemically processed? If so, note the type of service—perm, relaxer, two-step perm, color or bleach and the specific type of product, such as permanent color or henna.

If you have performed a chemical service on the client, reanalyze the hair in every category after the service. Porosity and tensile strength are the most likely to have changed.

The best time to gather further information is while you are styling the client's hair. First inquire about mechanical influences. Ask the client how he or she prefers to style the hair at home and which tools and brushes or combs are used. If your client uses thermal tools, you'll want to recommend a thermal protector and conditioner. The specific recommendation will be further narrowed, based on the hair type, condition and previous service.

Next discuss the client's styling routine. Lifestyle should have been explored prior to delivering the service in order to arrive at a service decision. (You wouldn't give a client who leads a hectic lifestyle a hairstyle that requires time-consuming, daily upkeep.) Now delve deeper by asking which styling products your client is most comfortable using. Some clients prefer two-in-one shampoo/conditioners; others are familiar with gels but are less comfortable using mousses or pomades. If your client is unfamiliar with the styling product that you know is most appropriate, determine whether the client is open to learning how to use the product.

The results of the hair analysis and the client's answers to each question will help you decide which personalized hair-care program you will recommend.

Based on the total picture, recommend a shampoo, conditioner and daily styling products. Use the following general guidelines to mix and match recommendations. (What follows are just some of the possibilities.)

FINE, LIMP HAIR

◆ Body-building shampoo
◆ Light conditioner, to be used on the ends only if hair tends to get limper from conditioners

- Hair-thickening products
- Hairsprays
- Bodifying gels and mousses

COARSE, RESISTANT HAIR

- Moisturizing shampoo or shampoo for dry hair
- Cream conditioner to improve combability
- Strong-hold sculpting gel with conditioners
- Styling spritzes for strong root lift

WAVY, DRY HAIR

- Moisture-balanced, pH-balanced shampoo
- Moisturizing conditioner
- Alcohol-free mousse
- Pomades and sculpting gel for styling shape into hair
- Pomades

HAIR THAT WILL BE HEAT-STYLED

- Protein shampoo
- Reconstructive conditioner
- Thermal protector
- Leave-in conditioner with sunscreen
- Alcohol-free styling products, including blow-drying lotion and light pressing cream or oil if hair will be pressed
- Shampoos that remove product buildup, for use once a week
- Pomades and shine enhancers
- Light hair dressings, silicone sealers for iron curled styles

BRAIDED STYLES

- Moisturizing shampoos and conditioners, formulated for braided hair
- Braid oil
- Scalp oils (avoid greasy, oily products)
- Scalp cleansers, including cholesterol

CHEMICALLY TREATED HAIR BY TYPE OF SERVICE

Relaxed or Texturized

- Neutralizing shampoo after the service; pH-balanced, moisturizing shampoo for dry hair at home
- Instant conditioner or leave-in conditioners
- Deep conditioner/remoisturizer
- Styling sprays that minimize damage from thermal styling
- Light oil sheen spray
- Avoid thick, greasy conditioners that could harden on hair, and do not overuse protein products

◆ Avoid overly oily products and shampoos for oily hair

Permed in Two Steps

- ◆ Shampoo for chemically treated hair
- ◆ Instant conditioners or leave-in conditioners
- ◆ Remoisturizing deep conditioner
- ◆ Curl activator to restore curl pattern
- ◆ Oil sheen spray to restore shine
- ◆ Humectants and glycerin products
- ◆ Light gels
- ◆ Avoid products that contain alcohol, shampoos for oily hair and products that stiffen or harden on the hair. Don't overuse activators to conceal a procedure gone wrong.

Permed in a Single Step

- ◆ Shampoo for permed hair; moisturizing shampoo
- ◆ Conditioner formulated for hair strengthening, body-building
- ◆ Protein treatments
- ◆ Curl rejuvenators, alcohol-free mousses
- ◆ Avoid products that contain alcohol

Color Treated or Bleached

- ◆ Moisturizing shampoo or shampoo for dry hair
- ◆ Color-enhancing shampoos
- ◆ Conditioners formulated to protect haircolor
- ◆ Leave-in conditioners with sunscreen
- ◆ Alcohol-free stying products that contain panthenol, sunscreens
- ◆ Avoid shampoos that remove buildup unless the manufacturer specifically states that they will not affect haircolor.

PRESCRIPTIVE PARTNERSHIPS

Once you know the type of products that you will prescribe to a client based on a complete analysis of the situation, the simplest way to retail is to make the client your partner in the decision. During the retail consultation, keep in mind that each product should be presented in terms of its features and the benefit of those features to the client. For example, a feature of a product is that it contains sunscreen; the benefit to the client is that it will prevent haircolor from fading, make it possible to stretch out color appointments (if necessary) and extend service dollars, giving the client more value.

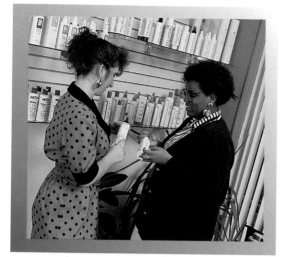

FIGURE 18.1
Make the client part of the consultation and part of the decisionmaking. Photo: Michael Gallitelli on location at Rielms Hair Salon, Latham, New York.

A simple way to make the client your partner is to elicit his or her opinions, likes and dislikes. The following six steps, which can be combined in any way, provide a foundation for partnership selling.

1. **Ask the client basic questions that ultimately relate to product usage.** Determine the client's likes and dislikes about styling, just as before the service you asked about likes and dislikes relating to a cut or chemical service. Determine if the client knows how to maintain the service received. If a client who got a two-step perm is planning to use a variety of thermal styling techniques, the client the perm will be weakened.

2. **Ask more concise questions about the types of products the client currently uses.** By doing this, you will narrow down the client's the needs and wants further. For example, if the client wants volume and doesn't feel comfortable using mousses, a gel—used at the base of the hair shaft for lift—may be the retail solution.

3. **Come to a conclusion based on the client's answers.** The answers to your questions will direct you to the proper prescriptive retail products. Perhaps a client will not be satisfied unless the hair feels soft after styling or only wants products that add shine.

4. **Reiterate what you heard.** Here, repeat to the client what you heard the client say about his or her needs or wants. Make certain you're speaking the same language. For example, say, "What you're saying is that you prefer a gel, but you want one that adds shine and won't build up."

5. **Make a suggestion.** Pair the client's needs and wants with specific products that your salon carries. If the client hates lack of volume, doesn't like to use hairspray and wants shine, select a styling product that delivers what's needed and is formulated for the client's hair type and/or the service just delivered.

6. **Get the client's input.** Don't just wait to be turned down after suggesting a product; tell the client you'd like him or her to see the item and give you feedback. If the client has an objection, reframe the objection as a question. For example, you suggested a gel but the client thinks gels are sticky and stiff. Ask, "If you could find a gel that gave your hair volume and kept it feeling soft, would you try it?" This is a technique used by salespeople in every industry.

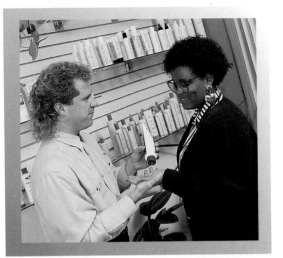

FIGURE 18.2
Let the client feel and smell the product. Get it into the client's hands. Photo: Michael Gallitelli on location at Rielms Hair Salon, Latham, New York.

At this point you should place the specific product in the client's hands. Let the client smell the product, read the ingredients label and try it out. Getting a product into the client's hands is called "ownership," and several studies have shown that if you can get the client to touch and feel a product, the client is twice as likely to purchase it. If the client is still uncertain, offer a product sample. Sampling is one of the most overlooked techniques of successful prescriptive retailing. In one study, over half the clients who sampled a product returned to purchase it.

Prior to using the six steps to partnership selling with a client, role-play with another stylist. Take turns playing client. This way you will become much more comfortable with applying the steps in the salon. If any step seems unnatural to you, make adjustments based on what feels right to you. You cannot retail effectively if you sound like you're reading lines out of a book.

SAMPLE SOUND BITES

The next time you go to a department store, purchase an item by mail order—or shop around and eavesdrop on salespeople and customers—pay attention to the language used or the dialogue you hear. Does the salesperson sound insincere and only interested in making a sale, or is the salesperson discussing the customer's needs? Are features and benefits of the product mentioned? Does the salesperson make the item sound exciting? By analyzing sales conversations, you'll quickly become sensitive to what is in the customer's interest and what is simply a "sales pitch."

Never try to sell an item simply to make a sale. In the cosmetology profession, this is completely unnecessary because almost everyone needs and uses shampoos, conditioners and styling products. By making a professional recommendation, you help your client narrow the confusing array of choices available today.

The following sample "sound bites" are tailored toward the client who has just received a relaxing service. Examples are given for opening sentences, describing feature/benefits of a product and responding to a client's needs and/or objections.

Opening Sentences

"Relaxed hair tends to get dry; did you notice that last time you had your hair relaxed?"

"How do you like to style your hair at home?"

"Which shampoos and conditioners do you use at home? (Wait for answer) Do you know if they're slightly acid or alkaline? (Wait for answer) The reason I ask is because relaxers are alkaline, and if you use a shampoo and conditioner that's slightly acidic, it counteracts the alkalinity, so your hair and scalp maintain their natural balance."

Feature/Benefit Descriptions

"I noticed your hair is a little dry. We just got a new conditioner that has panthenol, aloe vera, collagen and Vitamins A, B, D and E in it, which all prevent your hair from looking and feeling dry. I'm going to use it on your hair now, and you can feel it when I'm done styling it."

"If you're going to set your hair, I have the perfect thing for you. This setting lotion doesn't contain any alcohol, so it won't make your hair drier. It's not sticky at all; put a little in your hand and feel it."

"See how shiny your hair looks now? This moisturizer will help keep it that way. (Show client product) It's what we used today. It has all natural botanicals in it, so you won't be adding more chemicals to your hair."

Responses to Needs and Objections

"You said you want your hair to feel soft. This is what I used today. Now, feel your hair."

"If you could find a shampoo with a conditioner right in it, would you like that better than having to take the time to use both? (For the client who indicated a streamlined hair-care program was desirable.)

"OK, you have plenty of shampoo right now, but I'm going to give you this sample to use because it'll really help your hair right after it's been relaxed, and I want your hair to keep looking as great as it does now. It keeps your hair from getting too dry because it has panthenol in it, and it's really gentle. Use it for the next week and let me know what you think."

"It does cost a little more, but I've found that most conditioners have too much protein in them for relaxed hair. Protein can make relaxed hair drier and make it feel hard. This is actually a moisturizer and you only use this much (show the client), so it only costs a few cents every time you use it. It'll lubricate your hair and your scalp and you can even apply just a little to your scalp if it feels dry. I'll show you how."

EDUCATION: THE COMPELLING FOUNDATION

In the previous examples, professional education is the foundation for the "whys and hows" that you tell a client. If you understand all hair types and the chemistry of services, you'll be able to rely on this knowledge when prescribing retail.

You'll have to pair this knowledge with product knowledge. Don't be tempted to skip manufacturer's product knowledge classes; demand more. Ask questions about ingredients. Today's consumers are ingredient-savvy, and a salon owner may want to invest in a cosmetic ingredients dictionary for the entire salon. If not, many manufacturers will provide you with information on the ingredients in their specific product lines.

Always rely on a sound educational foundation, not on "selling tricks." While some books suggest "mirroring," which means acting as a mirror by imitating the client's body posture, many people are aware of this trick, and you'd look awfully silly making a face if the client is doing so.

Incidentally, do observe body posture and facial expressions—don't ignore them. If the client seems to be displeased, encourage honest feedback. Women might love an aromatherapy shampoo; a man might make a face when you show him the bottle because he considers the scent too feminine.

A WORD ABOUT PRODUCT SELECTION

Unless you are the salon owner or an independent contractor, you won't have a lot of say about the product lines your salon carries. Some owners ask senior stylists to test a new line before adding it in the salon; others carry seven to ten lines to satisfy walk-in customers who are drawn by national advertising.

Let the owner know that you want to retail and that you understand it's an important part of the service. If the salon carries ten lines, familiarize yourself with all of them so you can make the appropriate suggestion. Sometimes the primary difference will be price point. If you know price is important to the client, narrow your suggestions on this basis.

Any salon that is interested in doing business in the future will carry lines for several markets. Men prefer simple packaging in dark or neutral colors. Hispanics prefer products that have instructions in Spanish. African Americans want a line that is especially targeted at them.

In general, everyone likes something that seems like it is especially for them. This is why shampoos and conditioners that were formulated for color-treated and permed hair have received so much acceptance. The customer thinks, "This was created just for me," and, in fact, it was.

PRODUCT DISPLAYS

Today many business owners are more open to suggestions that come from the bottom up, thanks to a new approach to management, which has eliminated hierarchal layers and recognizes that the front-line person knows the most about how to improve the job—and customer service. Salons have always been more entrepreneurial than corporations; therefore, the more you know about business, the better. Whether you want to own your own salon some day or want to take on the responsibility of creating retail displays to further your career, the following guidelines will help you create displays that are practically self-selling:

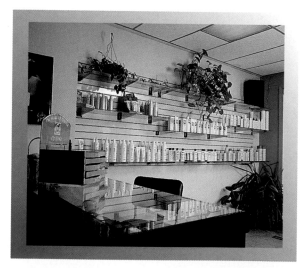

FIGURE 18.3
Retail displays should be inviting. Be sure your clients can touch, feel and smell the products. Photo: Michael Gallitelli on location at Rielms Hair Salon, Latham, New York.

◆ Retail displays should invite the customer to touch, feel and smell. Don't hide products behind counters, or that's where they'll stay. Display products in attractive baskets and add dried flowers. Open up one or two and label them as samplers. Take a walk through free-standing stores, such as The Body Shop or H_2O, and you'll get a feel for displays that encourage "ownership."

◆ If you use large displays, set them up to follow the same pattern the eye does when it scans. (Maggie McCain-Davis was the first to pioneer this approach in the salon industry.) The eye moves from the high left to the lower right, because this is how we read. Place weight or your largest items on the bottom of a display and the eye will travel back up once it hits this optical weight line. On each shelf, position the largest size at the far right, the next largest size adjacent to it, and so forth. Largest sizes go on the right because most people reach from right to left. Place best-selling items at eye level; organize types of products horizontally so that all shampoos create one horizontal line, all gels create

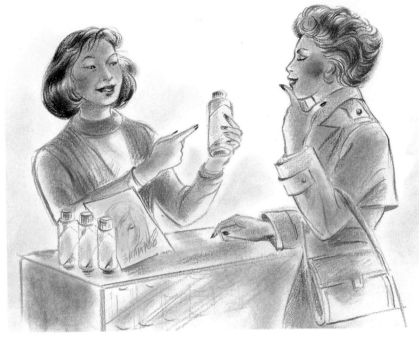

FIGURE 18.4
Retailing to multicultural clients.

another, and so on. Of course, if your primary clientele are native readers of Chinese, Japanese, Korean or other similar languages, their natural scanning pattern will move from top to bottom. If this is the case, familiarize yourself with the specific language and how it is read.

◆ If you use shelving, stock products about four deep and create two or three horizontal rows of shampoo from a single product line before adding a shampoo from the next product line. (Remember, largest one first, on the far right.)

◆ Use mirrors behind wall shelves to create the illusion of more product.

◆ Place displays within the first ten feet of the salon.

◆ Use free-standing mini displays throughout the salon. These displays are fun to create, and you can design them using the same principles that you use to create a balanced hair design.

◆ Always display prices and add signs, but don't clutter displays. Prices can be displayed on stickers that are placed on bottles.

◆ If you create a display that results in a sales increase, it's a good argument for a bonus or a new area of responsibility, such as visual merchandising.

PRODUCT PRICING

The savvy stylist should understand product pricing and the language of retail. We are, if anything, a nation of middlemen. Manufacturers, distributors and salon owners all get a cut before the stylist, which narrows your personal profit while increasing the cost to the client. If a salon carries a private label product, the distributor is eliminated; therefore the salon makes more profit on the item. The trade-off is that you lose the support of national advertising and other such programs that will draw the client to the product.

The most commonly used retail terms are the following:

Mark-up. All salon owners want to pay less for product than they sell it for. Mark-up is the profit a salon wants to make, or the discount at which the salon wants to buy the product. If you want a 50 percent discount—or a 50 percent profit, add 50 percent mark-up to the cost to set the client's cost.

Discount. This is the difference between the client's price and the salon's cost, expressed as percentage. It's also the percent you want to make. You will often hear distributors discussing a 50 percent or 40 percent line. Private label products are often 100 percent lines.

Margin. The margin is the difference between the price at which you sell a product and how much you paid for it. The margin is gross profit to the salon before the stylist is paid commission or other deductions are taken to fund benefits plans or overhead, or anything else that the salon owner has determined that retail will finance.

Turnover. This is the rate at which products or the salon's retail inventory is sold, expressed as a yearly rate. If a case of a particular hairspray has a 6X turnover rate, this means that the inventory of hairspray sells out six times a year, or every two months. Products with high turnover are best sellers. If items have a low turnover, the salon may want to drop the line or order less of the item, if it is popular with a core of customers but not a hot seller.

GOAL SETTING

If you understand the above terminology, it will become clear why salons rarely pay a stylist more than 10 to 15 percent commission on retail sales. If salons are using retail sales to fund other programs, such as health care, a 401k fund, advertising and promotion, or a bonus program, owners may pay as little as 5 percent. However, by using a prescriptive partnership approach to retailing you should be able to add 200 dollars or more to your monthly income, even at the lowest rate of commission.

Stylists who make significant money retailing are prescribing the correct products for all their clients and are setting retail goals. When setting goals, don't fall into the trap of setting simple dollar goals. The most successful retailers set goals in terms of percentage of clients who rely on their professional advice.

IN THE MIX

The salon that builds a multicultural clientele is the most likely to have a significant retailing business in the future—if the salon is dedicated to retail. This is not only due to changing demographics, but because certain segments of the market, such as African Americans, spend more money on hair-care products than other segments do.

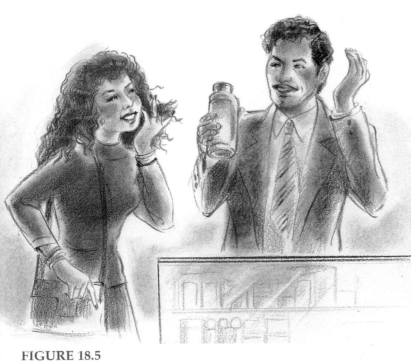

FIGURE 18.5
Retailing.

Some products act as "crossover" products, and some lines are even marketed this way. However, keep in mind that many clients prefer products that are marketed specifically for them and their hair. While some salons say they make no special effort because they naturally service all clients, the clients may not be getting that message.

Relaxed hair, braided hair and hair that has been permed in two steps has its own special needs, and many product lines are created to meet them. Arranging these retail products in a prominent window display is one of the quickest ways to let passers-by know that your salon serves all clients. Familiarize yourself with all these products so that you can make the very best prescriptive retail suggestions.

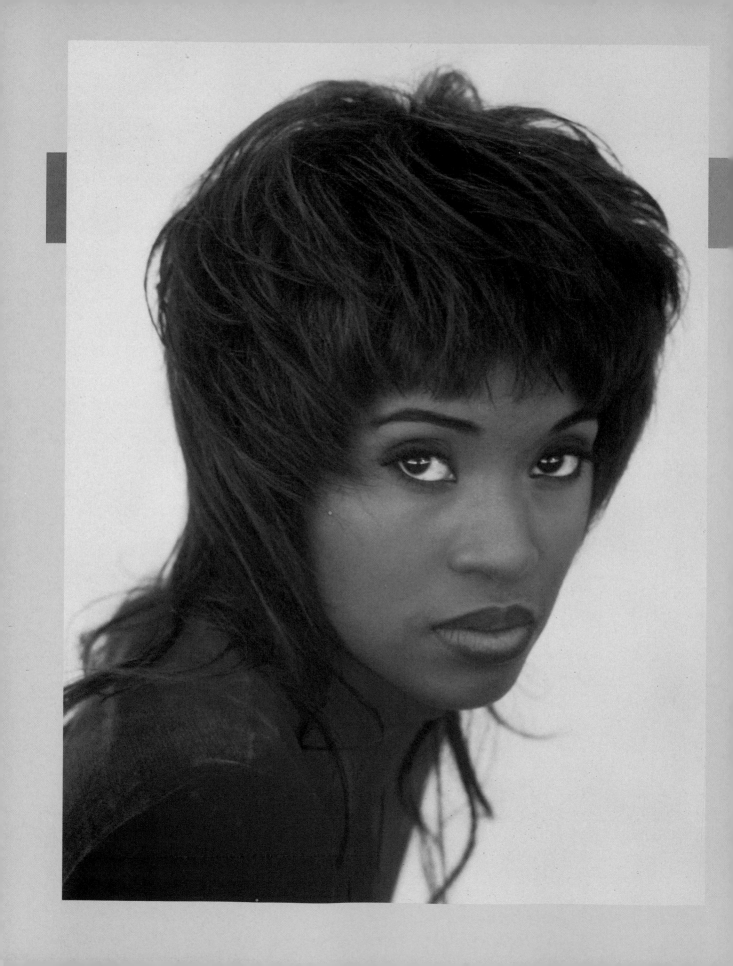

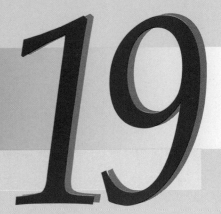

Chapter 19

Building a Career

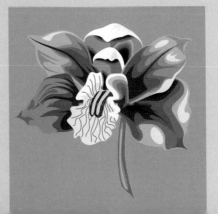

Understanding how to work with all types of hair is just one way to build a career for the future. In his book *New Work Habits for a Radically Changing World,* Price Pritchett notes that taking care of a career today means managing perpetual motion. And the key to success is taking personal responsibility for growth when businesses are undergoing rapid change. In other words, today's stylists have to think like business owners.

Just a few of the changes salons are undergoing are the move toward a part-time work force, a rapid increase in independent contractors, growth that lies with chains more than independent salons, a shortage of stylists, the move toward self-managing teams within the salon and operational changes due to new technology. As with many other businesses, there's no longer any such thing as job security in the salon.

This chapter will help you build your business, take responsibility for your own career and grow with a changing market into the twenty-first century. If you're well-educated and working in a service business, you're in a position to succeed.

ATTRACTING A CLIENTELE

While salon owners can run ads and promotions to attract new clients, most frequently rely on the staff to attract and retain business. Most salon owners are open to suggestions and will support your efforts—sometimes with a financial investment in your idea.

While stylists are building new business, owners will refer new clients to them on a rotating business. This rarely grows your business as fast as you'd like. To build your book faster, take responsibility for attracting new clients by experimenting with the following ideas.

◆ Ask the owner to supply you with business cards. Pass them out to anyone and everyone and let them know you'd like to do their hair. Add a few tantalizing suggestions. If the owner agrees, you can offer a one-time discount to new clients. For example, if you're in a restaurant, in addition to a tip leave your business card marked "20 percent off any new service."

◆ Seek out employees who are highly visible, such as bank tellers, supermarket clerks, cosmetic counter people and retail salespeople. If you have lots of unscheduled booking time, offer to do their hair for 50 percent off or even for free if they will tell anyone who asks that you are their stylist. This technique has worked well for manicurists and estheticians, as well as hairstylists.

◆ Offer your clients a reward for referrals. Give clients five of your business cards with the client's name written on the back. When five referrals come in with one person's name, give that client one free service.

◆ Seek out places on your own where potential clients can be found. For instance, if you have a local weight-loss center, ask the owner to tell clients that once they reach their halfway goal, you'll give them a new cut or style at 50 percent off and once they achieve their total goal, you'll provide a complete makeover to work with their fabulous new look.

◆ Tap niches. Teens, business women, men, mature clients, Asians, Latinos, African Americans, nursing home residents and fledgling models all represent market niches that you can tap. While some salons simply say they serve everyone, this does not ensure attracting a diverse clientele. Based on the population of your geographic area, target a particular market niche, go where its members are and try to attract them to your salon. For this to succeed, the targeted group should live reasonably close to your salon. If the only modeling agency is ten miles from your salon, you might not be as successful as the stylist whose salon is next door. Develop a creative promotion, offer clients services in return for permission to take and use "before" and "after" photos and invent new styles that appeal to the group you're targeting. If you want to reach the youth market, go to local clubs wearing a hot new style, or get a "club kid" to do it for you.

◆ If you are new at a salon, talk to the owner about promoting you. Make it clear you'll be promoting yourself in various ways, and ask for assistance. Owners will post your name in the window; some will even run a local ad announcing the fact you've joined the salon.

◆ Take part in community events and fundraisers. Join local clubs. The more you support your community, the more visible you'll become, and the more the community will support you.

RETAINING NEW CLIENTS

Your income depends on your ability to keep new clients, and salons often give raises that are partly based on a stylist's retention rate. In several surveys, clients indicated they would travel farther to patronize a business that provided superior customer service, and "service" goes far beyond your cutting, styling and chemical service skills.

To offer your clients the service they want, and keep them coming to you, follow these suggestions for retaining clients:

◆ Schedule extra time for every first-time consultation. Concentrate on listening to clients' desires, repeating back what you heard and performing an analysis-based consultation. Always give a reason for a suggestion that relates to the client's desires.

◆ Even though you want to build business fast, avoid over-booking. There's nothing worse than rushing a first-time client or keeping a client waiting.

◆ Go the extra mile. Show clients how to style their new look and give them as many tips as possible that relate to hair care. Avoid gossiping, beyond establishing a rapport. Use your time with the client to give him or her something special.

◆ While you work, give the client something to think about for the next appointment. Say, "Your hair would look terrific with just a few highlights around the face. Why don't you think about doing them next time?" Sometimes the client shows enough interest that you can add the service that day.

◆ When the client leaves, hand the person your business card and say, "Feel free to call me if you have any trouble styling your hair or if you have any questions at all."

◆ Call the client a few days after the service to inquire about how the new style is working out. This is particularly important with chemical-service clients. If the client indicates there is any problem at all, immediately invite the client back for a free consultation or to fix a problem.

◆ Maintain your professional poise and your service attitude at all times. The client is always right, because the client is the one who has to live with a new look. Even when someone wants something that's not your personal taste, adapt to the client's personal style preferences.

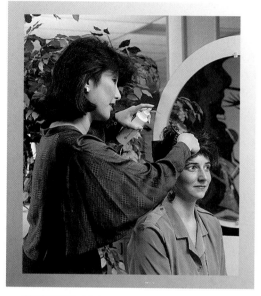

FIGURE 19.1
Show clients how to create their style. Photo: Michael Gallitelli on location at Rielms Hair Salon, Latham, New York.

REBOOKING STRATEGIES

If you keep detailed client record cards, getting clients to rebook is easier. Salons that are computerized can easily locate and contact clients who are due for a service; if the salon is not computerized, develop a rotating filing system so that the cards of clients who have not come in for six months will stand out.

Ask the salon owner if there is a policy regarding reminder cards. Some salons send them regularly to chemical-service clients or mail service-discount offers to clients who have not returned to the salon for six months. If the salon has no standing policy, ask the owner if you can be responsible for this. Even if you pay your own postage to send out personalized postcards or call clients yourself, the effort is worth the cost, which may be tax deductible.

Some salons are uncomfortable about allowing stylists access to client files; others have a written policy that the clients belong to the salon, not the individual. Still others ask stylists to sign a non-compete agreement before hiring, which states that clients cannot be contacted by the stylist. Unless you really want the job, avoid signing employee contracts.

If you cannot gain an owner's trust, offer to write out postcards to clients and let the salon mail them.

All of these tactics are after the fact; the simplest way to get clients to rebook is to do it before they leave the salon. Let them know when they will be due for a retouch or a trim, and ask if they'd like to book that appointment before they leave. Let them know that they can always change the appointment if necessary.

Businesses such as dental offices excel in this approach. If the client doesn't book before he or she leaves, the office sends reminder cards and follows up with a phone call. Their booking and retention rates are extremely high, with some that use this system operating at 98 percent retention.

If you suspect a client is not returning because of a problem, call the client—or have the salon owner call—and say you've noticed the client has not been in for some time. Then ask if the client was unhappy with the last service, and be prepared to set your ego aside and listen. You may not like what you hear, but you'll learn something useful for the future.

SPECIALIZING IN THE SALON

Many specialities are open to the advanced stylist who wants to hone skills in a particular area. Manicuring and esthetics are the traditional separate paths cosmetologists can take; newer specializations include colorist, natural hair-care specialist, hair-replacement specialist, chemical specialist and makeup artist. In addition, those who specialize find other doors are open, such as educator, platform artist and consultant.

To specialize in any area, take advanced education classes, read everything you can about your chosen area and network with other professionals. Locating a mentor who already specializes in your chosen area is a sure way to learn all you can and climb a career path.

If you think specializing might be right for you, read the following brief descriptions of each specialization. Descriptions include a look at future growth and tips from professionals who already specialize.

HAIR COLORIST

Many salons have created separate color departments, making it easy for you to locate a position in which you can specialize in haircolor. Colorists can charge more for their services than stylists, and corrective colorists are in high demand.

Once you locate a salon that has color specialists, contact the owner, let him or her know what your career plans are and request a meeting to obtain professional advice. It's rare you'll be turned down. Be prepared to explain your interest in color, lay out your plans for obtaining advanced education and ask the owner about color apprenticeships. Frequently salons that do not have official job openings will take you on as an apprentice if they are impressed with your desire to learn.

Trade shows that emphasize haircolor, such as Haircolor USA and the Haircolor Exchange, are excellent places to learn and network. You can locate them in the trade show event listings of professional publications, such as *Modern Salon* magazine (Lincolnshire, Ilinois) and *Shoptalk* (Chicago, Illinois).

The more advanced classes you can take through a manufacturer or distributor, the more likely you are to secure an apprenticeship, meet important contacts and build your color education. It's also a good idea to invest in a mannequin head and test several different product lines on it, to familiarize yourself with subtle differences in products.

In the salon, apprentices start out assisting with applications and foiling, but the opportunity to learn more about formulation is always present. Often the salon will provide additional education during training nights.

Colorists work closely with hair designers to create total looks. Your ability to work in harmony with others and create color effects that enhance a specific haircut is important. The Minardi Beauty Focus, held in New York through Minardi Salon, is an ideal place to learn how cut and color work together and receive advanced color education.

With advanced education and experience, you can progress from apprentice, to colorist, to department head, to educator or platform artist. The future for colorists is very bright. Factors that contribute to the growth in haircolor are the graying of America, a tremendous increase in demand for haircolor in the African American and Hispanic markets, and new, gentler products that appeal to all clients, including the formerly color-shy.

CHEMICAL SPECIALIST

While it's rare for a salon have a separate perming department, many have separate chemical-service areas, in which perming, relaxing and coloring take place. These are the big ticket services, so specializing in them will boost your income considerably. Even if the salon you're in takes an "everyone does it all" approach, you can tell the owner you'd like to specialize in chemical services, build your educational background and promote yourself that way. If your business and reputation take off, you could end up with your own area in the salon or with trainees working under you.

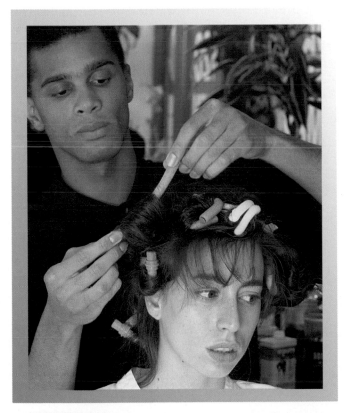

FIGURE 19.2
Become a chemical specialist. Photo: Steven Landis with direction from Vincent and Alfred Nardi of Nardi Salon, New York City, New York.

The skills needed to specialize are different than those required to be a great haircutter. If your ability to cut and style or "move" hair is adequate but not outstanding—and you like details, such as chemistry and information about hair structure—specializing in chemical services might be right for you. Stylists who are excellent haircutters are not necessarily terrific at delivering chemical services, as consumer magazine articles about bad perming experiences attest.

Manufacturers and distributors offer ample education in chemical services, and attendance at most trade shows will help you increase your knowledge. A basic chemistry course at a local university or college will also give you a solid foundation on which to build.

Specializing in chemical services puts you in a position for career longevity. Perhaps you've heard, "When color-service sales are up, perm sales are down." This is almost always true. However, if you can deliver both, and if you understand relaxing and two-step perms, the economy, demographic changes and new trends will never adversely affect your business. You'll simply deliver more of one service than another at different points in your career.

NATURAL HAIR CARE SPECIALIST

While only New York State currently offers a separate license in natural hair care, the movement toward separate licensing is growing fast. The best place to learn and practice this art is in large metropolitan areas with diverse populations.

The natural hair care specialist does not work with chemicals or thermal tools, but practices a totally natural approach to hair care, maintenance and styling. Knowledge of braiding and hair addition services is essential.

If you have had problems with allergic reactions to products in the past, natural hair care provides an excellent opportunity to continue to practice your craft.

If you cannot locate a salon in which to apprentice in your area, contact the National Braiders Network, located in Brooklyn, New York, and ask for a local referral. If there are no salons in your area, you'll have to travel to learn more, but if you already have a cosmetology license and add these skills to your repertoire, you could be the first person in your area to offer natural hair care. You'll be able to practice because you already have the state required cosmetology license; as more states add a specialty license, it's likely that you'll be qualified to obtain one if you took the New York State course.

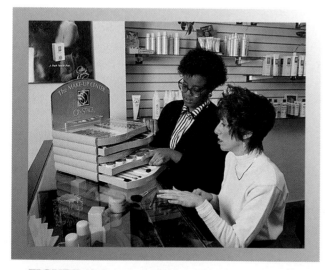

FIGURE 19.3
Makeup artistry is an exciting, challenging career. Photo: Michael Gallitelli on location at Rielms Hair Salon, Latham, New York.

MAKEUP ARTIST

In salons, makeup artists are frequently freelancers or independent contractors who set their own hours. If you like makeup and have an entrepreneurial, independent spirit, this specialty can take you far. However, you must be prepared for the reality that, in salons, the money is in the sale of take-home products, not in the delivery of the service. Often makeup lessons and makeup touch-ups are offered on a complimentary basis. So you'd better like selling.

The markup on makeup and cosmetics is usually 100 percent and the average ticket in many department stores is close to 300 dollars. Out-marketing the department stores is key for success in the salon. The average salon ticket is lower than that of department stores, but salons that use department store display and merchandising concepts find they can easily make an excellent living, working part-time.

To specialize in makeup, sign up for manufacturer classes and consider attending a special makeup school, such as the Westmore Academy in Los Angeles. Take marketing and merchandising class-

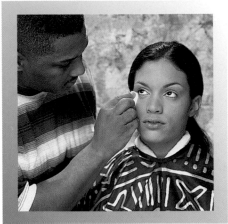

FIGURE 19.4
Makeup artistry.

es at your local university and frequently visit department, specialty and free-standing stores to observe their displays and merchandising approaches. Ample stock and attractive displays that invite the customer to touch and feel are essential to sales success.

Once you build your skills, you can move beyond the salon, where the service itself becomes more important. Ask new photographers if you can do makeup for their models for free in return for photos for your portfolio. As you build your portfolio, you'll be able to show it to photographers, magazines and advertising agencies and secure jobs as an editorial and advertising makeup artist or even as a film makeup artist. (The latter requires acceptance in a union.)

Related areas include paramedical makeup artist, camouflage makeup artist and special-effects makeup artist. These all require special training and a particular disposition. Working in a burn unit of a hospital or having the patience to spend long hours on a movie set are not for everyone, but if it does suit you, they represent some of the most rewarding careers possible within this specialty.

HAIR-REPLACEMENT SPECIALIST

By now you've heard enough about the aging of the population to know that any service that helps people stay youthful-looking, healthy and fit will be in increased demand in the next ten to thirty

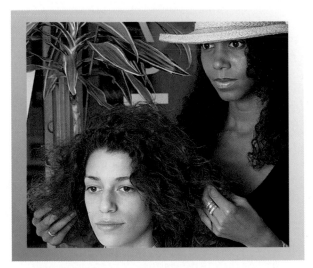

FIGURE 19.5
Client consultation should be a big part of your cosmetology career. Photo: Michael Gallitelli on location at Rielms Hair Salon, Latham, New York.

years. Hair loss is one of the most cosmetically distressing aspects of aging, and youth-oriented baby boomers are certain to do all they can to prevent hair loss and camouflage it when it occurs. The average consumer is unaware of the options available and will be delighted to find a professional who is well-versed in hair-loss solutions.

The primary stumbling block to specializing in this area is that training is not as readily available as it is for other specialities. Hair replacement centers protect their techniques as though they were national-security secrets, because the company's goal is to convince you to buy a franchise. While this may be an option, you should investigate any company thoroughly before making such an investment.

Many of the non-surgical, natural-looking techniques involve some form of bonding. Individual hairs are attached to existing ones and bonded in

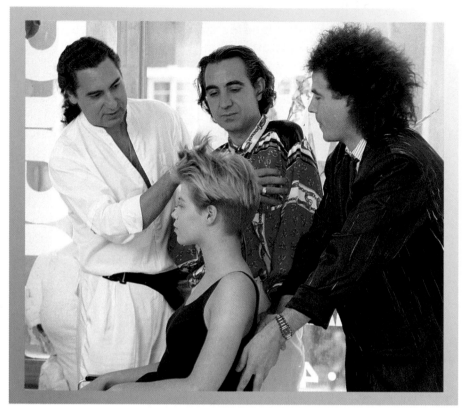

FIGURE 19.6
Consultations. Photo: Michael Gallitelli on location at Rielms Hair Salon, Latham, New York.

place. Usually the service is delivered in a series because the hair is attached in rows. After the first few are formed and hairs are anchored to the natural hair, subsequent hairs are attached to the new "implants," as more rows of hair are created. (While replacement centers frequently use the word "implant" to communicate permanency, the hair is technically not an implant since it is not added surgically.) Other popular techniques rely on custom-made systems, which are similar to integration systems. They are based on hand-knotting hair to very light webbing or "breathable skin" bases, which are then woven into the hair.

Hair replacement centers charge thousands of dollars for their painstaking work, and their fees are out of the range of many clients. In the salon, you can offer alternatives, such as hair additions and hair integration systems, depending on the degree of hair loss.

To increase your skills in this area, contact manufacturers of toupees, integration systems and wigs and ask about advanced education classes. The National Cosmetology Association (NCA), headquartered in St. Louis, Misouri, supports the "Look Good/Feel Better" program, which involves salons assisting chemotherapy patients, and can put you in touch with specialists who help these clients cosmetically conceal temporary hair loss. In addition, European schools and manufacturers of hair wefts offer advanced education in hair replacement.

Through the NCA or your local yellow pages, you may be able to locate a salon in your area where you can apprentice. This is one of the best ways to learn because hands-on experience is essential. If you are working elsewhere, you might offer to apprentice or pay for training one or two nights a week. Masters of this profession enjoy passing on their knowledge, and their years of experience will be invaluable to you. In addition, established braiders often know techniques for attaching hair additions when only a sparse amount of natural hair remains. If you attend a trade show targeted at the African-American or Hispanic market, you'll get the opportunity to network with braiders and hair manufacturers, who often offer classes at these shows.

Once your skills are established, you'll have to target a clientele. Work with your local American Cancer Society, hospitals, nursing homes, women's clubs, men's health clubs and any business where the over-forty crowd gathers. Offer to create tie-in promotions, give free seminars or demonstrate your skills. Local advertising that positions you as a specialist is also worth paying for, since you want to attract specific clients. Ask any magazine or newspaper in which you are considering running an advertisement which sections have the highest forty-plus readership, and request that your ad be positioned there. Often an ad positioned in the business pages or sports section will reach the clients you want to attract most.

This is a service that is sorely lacking in many areas. If you can be the first to specialize, you may find that local papers will be very interested in writing a story about you, and local television appearances may not be difficult to secure. Contact the producer of the show on which you want to appear, and send a letter detailing your speciality, along with before and after photos of your work. Offer to appear on the show, and suggest a segment that has a particular slant to it, such as, "Ways to look great on your 50th birthday." Needless to say, you wouldn't approach a youth-oriented show with this idea. For that market, suggest a segment on "Fun with hairpieces" or "How you can look like a famous rock singer," and demonstrate your skills with hair additions.

HOW TO KNOW WHEN IT'S TIME TO MOVE ON

Stylists are notorious for salon hopping for a higher commission, but this is no way to build a career. As long as the salon in which you work offers an opportunity to learn and grow, it's worth staying to build a client base. However, if you are making an effort to learn, but are not, or if the owner isn't dedicated to helping you increase your professionalism, it may be time to move on.

If you find yourself thinking of leaving your current situation, ask yourself the following questions, to make certain the move is right for you.

1. Why am I thinking of leaving? Am I simply bored and not making the situation work, or is the salon in which I'm working wrong for me?

300 ◆ The Multicultural Client

2. Do I get fringe benefits, such as health insurance and profit sharing, at my current salon? As time passes, these will be increasingly important.

3. If I want a higher commission, am I booked at least 90 percent of the time where I am? If not, a higher commission isn't the key to growth. If you are booked 90 percent of the time, will the salon let you increase your prices so that you can make more with your current clientele?

4. Will the problem move with me? Not getting along with others, supervisors or more than one or two "problem" clients are situations that will reoccur unless you make adjustments in your approach to people. However, if the problem is with one key person who can affect your career, and you've tried to work it out to no avail, know when to cut your losses if the situation is so bad that you don't even want to go to work in the morning.

5. Where do I see myself in five years? In ten years? Is the salon in which I'm currently working helping put me on the track or impeding my progress?

6. Will a move to another salon allow me to develop a specialty, pay for advanced education or offer other special opportunities? Have I asked my current owner about offering those opportunities?

7. Am I ready to open my own business? Often stylists leave to open their own establishment without having learned the business aspects of running a salon. They take a few disgruntled staff members with them and try to start a new salon. After six months, they're in debt, working long hours behind the chair to make ends meet, and the disgruntled staff is now disgruntled with them. If you want to open your own salon, prepare by learning about marketing, finance, accounting and management. To make a business run well, you can't be working behind the chair every day. Your business ends up neglected, and you end up stressed and stretched to your limits. Read books, take classes, observe all business aspects of running a salon (such as compensation systems, working with suppliers and setting prices) and create a business plan before you quit your job and open a salon. Then try to leave on good terms. Your former employer will be worried or threatened, unless you discuss your decision frankly and without condemnation—and don't open up right across the street. Whenever possible, leave behind a friend with whom you can network as an equal.

After answering questions abut your desire to move on, make a list of the advantages and disadvantages of staying where you are and moving on. Then compare the lists and see which has more positive aspects. If you know where you want to go, this is easy; if you don't have a specific job offer or salon in mind, the unknown becomes a strong negative. You may be willing to take chances on yourself, and every new job contains some unknowns, but if you haven't investigated new salons, you could end up even worse off.

In the end, how you feel about your job and your co-workers is the best determinate. Follow the path that makes you the happiest.

INDEPENDENT CONTRACTING

Independent contracting is a fast-growing career option that has created much debate. Some say it detracts from the professionalism of the industry and is only a tax-evasion technique. Others say it's the easiest way to stop handing over 50 percent of every ticket to someone else. Whatever your feelings about contracting, it's here to say. Only two states have outlawed it, and these two might reverse the laws against independent contracting.

More than anything else, independent contracting is a tax issue. The "owner" becomes a landlord who must meet specific I.R.S. guidelines to avoid heavy penalties for not taking payroll deductions. The contractor must meet his or her own tax obligations, and the I.R.S. is currently looking at contractors very carefully. In addition, independent contractors (ICs) must carry their own liability insurance, have their own set of Material Safety Data Sheets (MSDSs) and take responsibility for advertising, promotion and other such matters. One important thing to keep in mind is that because you are not an employee, you are not qualified to receive workman's compensation or unemployment, should you need them.

If you think becoming an independent contractor is right for you, investigate all the legal aspects. Talk to the owner of a rental salon about the details, and talk other ICs. Then sit down and determine if it is as financially appealing as it truly seems. The following checklist should help you determine what your income might be as an IC. It is based on an estimate of the current clients you can reasonably expect to retain, what they pay for your services and the average expenses of an IC. Shop around for rental prices to get a good idea of what they are in your area before you proceed.

POTENTIAL INDEPENDENT CONTRACTOR'S CHECKLIST

1. Estimate your weekly or monthly income. To do this, divide clients by the services they receive (cut, perm, color, relaxer) and estimate the number of clients you will have in each service category. Then multiply the number of clients within each category that you'll see each week or month by your service price. Finally, add up all the service prices to arrive at an estimated monthly income. Add estimated tips at the end.

2. Determine your expenses by the month. First list your monthly rent. Then add supplies, which will be 5 to 8 percent of your service income. (Multiply service income by .05.) Experts recommend that you set aside 40 percent for taxes. So multiply your total monthly income by .4, and add this figure to the running total. Next add liability insurance (about 400 dollars, divided by 12). Add another 2 percent for telephone expenses and 3 to 5 percent for advertising and promotion. (Multiply your monthly income by .02 to get the first figure; multiply it by .03 or .05, depending on how much promotion you need, to get advertising figures.) Last, add any educational expenses and equipment costs. Plan on at least 500 dollars a year for continuing education. (Divide those figures by 12, since you are estimating monthly expenses.) When you're done, you'll have your monthly business expenses.

3. Determine your net monthly profit. To do this, subtract your expenses from your income. Is what's left enough on which to live? Don't think you can cheat on expenses and lower the figure in order to make it more attractive. You can't pretend realistic costs aren't there. If you've come up short—or if you got a negative number—build your clientele and work on increasing your prices while retaining current clients before you try the checklist again.

STAYING ON TOP

However you choose to manage your career, you should always be on the alert for two things: Changes in the market and changes in trends. In the global village in which we live today, trends can emerge from anywhere. Attend shows, read magazines, pay attention to street styles and travel whenever you can to identify emerging trends.

The market is affected by demographics, economics and even politics. Pay attention to what clients talk about and what they want. Take note of who your clients are—and who they aren't. If your salon is located in an area with lots of teenagers and none are coming to you it's a sign that one day you'll have a stagnant clientele. Make adjustments to appeal to new markets, and build for the future. If the trend is "cheap chic" or discount shopping and it's particularly popular with a particular group in your area, create a special off-price night to attract these clients without dropping your regular prices. Whenever you can attract new clients or meet the needs of a growing market, you're ensuring your professional future.

While hairdressers certainly want to sound professional and need to share a common language, it's also their job to get close to customers. In a service business, you must understand what your client wants, be able to communicate easily and use words the client understands. If you can't do this, you can't meet your clients' needs.

In the working world stylists often use one word with a client and another with other professionals. Sometimes stylists "talk down" to clients. Or stylists don't bother to explain what they're doing because they see no sense in telling the client, "I'm going to use the gray rods, wrap them off-base and create dropped-stem pin curls at the ends."

But clients are interested in what you're doing. They're most interested in what it will do for them, but they like explanations too. When their friends like their hair, they want to say more than, "He did this thing in the back where he twisted the hair but part of it was hanging down." This doesn't communicate very much and leaves both parties feeling silly.

Sometimes the terms used in salons reflect a move toward increased professionalism. Today no colorist tells a client "I'm going to dye your hair," yet only in the last five years has the word *dye* begun to disappear from consumer magazines. It is still extremely common to see the word *dye* in women's magazines and even more common to hear it being used. If a consumer says "haircolor" it usually reflects a successful attempt on the part of a salon to educate its clientele.

To add to the confusion, manufacturers like to invent their own marketing buzzwords. Everyone's got their own system of cutting and a name for it that they hope will set them apart. Other words are invented because of product manufacturing processes. The use of a level system and references to tone in haircolor relate to chemistry and provide a system for educating colorists that usually translates from one product line to another. Sometimes words become part of a common language; other times, they don't.

The result of all these factors is that stylists don't communicate with the same words among one another, let alone make sense to the client. Add a multicultural clientele, and the communication problem increases. What many hairdressers call a *perm* is a *relaxer* to African-American clients. To consumers, a *weave* is a weave; to purist professionals it is just one attachment technique used to add hair additions.

DEFIITIONS OF COMMONLY USED TERMS

The following definitions will not completely solve the clear-and-common language problem, especially for purists. They reflect a professional but client-centered language that will help you work with a multicultural clientele. Definitions include cross-references and interchangeable terms, so you don't have to search all over only to discover that two different words describe the same thing. The first word listed is the one that is most commonly used.

When you can communicate with all clients easily and professionally, you'll be as close to a worthwhile, universal language as you can get.

AFRICAN LOCKS

Since this phrase is old, historically, but relatively new to some hairstylists, it's easy to learn and use a positive, client-centered definition from the start. African locks are cultivated locks, intentionally encouraged to coil on their own. They appear coiled and controlled, compared to Rastafarian locks, which appear more matted. In either case, avoid the negative *dreadlocks*. In other words, stick to the word the market uses; avoid a European-imposed description. Sometimes you'll see *locks* spelled as *locs*; don't let it throw you. Different spellings reflect personal preference and marketing fun.

AMMONIUM THIOGLYCOLATE

This is a chemical ingredient in some relaxers. It acts as a straightening or reducing agent and is similar to chemicals used in perms. That's why hair that's been straightened with a thio product can then be curled with a thio-based perm, but hair can't be chemically curled if it was relaxed with a sodium hydroxide product. Sodium and thio aren't similar and are therefore not compatible. Since a client may have relaxed the hair at home, it's best to become familiar with which product lines contain which ingredients. Clients are most likely to tell you the brand name they used.

BASE CONTROL

The base is the area between partings on which a roller or pin curl sits; you also take partings when you use a curling iron or other tools. If a tool is on-base, it sits in the center of the partings; if it's off-base, it is off-center. When it's off-base, it's either closer to the top, or over-directed, or dropped closer to the bottom, or under-directed. Clients will most easily understand that you take large or small sections and direct the hair to move in a particular direction, either to give them a look with more lift and fullness or hair that's smoother at the scalp, or "roots."

BONDING

A method for attaching hair to the natural hair that uses a latex-based bonding agent. This word has real purpose; if you use the word *glue* the client is bound to react negatively. Explain you're using a special bonding product made for hair and how it works.

BOX BRAIDS

These are individual braids that hang free. In some regions of the country, they're also called Senegalese braids.

BRAIDING

A catch-all phrase for the many ways that natural hair or added hair can be intertwined. If you offer braiding services, you should be well-versed in all the types of braids that are popular in your geographic area. Specific names and techniques differ widely from region to region, so it's best to get local education first and learn more from there.

BRASS

To you, these are undesirable undertones that are visible after color fade off. To the client, it is generally red, warmth or a harsh gold. The common ground: they're undesirable to either one of you. If the client says she doesn't want to see red or brass, use photos to establish whether it's ash she wants, or a warm shade that isn't harsh or brassy.

BRICKLAY

A pattern used in perming or roller setting that looks precisely the way bricks are laid. Each horizontal row is staggered so that no roller is perfectly aligned with the one in front of it or behind it. If you want to discuss this pattern with the client, the simplest approach is to tell her you're staggering the rods or rollers so she won't see "splits" or lines in the hair, which you know as lines of demarcation. The pattern helps curls blend more naturally.

BULB

This is a club-shaped structure below the scalp that forms the lower part of the root.

CALCIUM HYDROXIDE

Calcium hydroxide is a chemical ingredient in a relaxer that uses activators. The most important thing to know is that these relaxers are not compatible with thio-based products.

CASAMAS

Very large braids are created by taking individual partings in any shape (square, triangular and so forth) and creating three-strand braids. The braids get their name from the fact that they were worn by the Casamas people in Senegal.

COLOR REMOVER

This is a product created specifically to remove haircolor from hair. Most contain bleach; therefore, they should never be used on relaxed hair. For safety's sake read all the directions and call the manufacturer's hotline if you have any questions.

CONTRIBUTING PIGMENT

The client's natural pigment must be considered when you color the hair, aiming for a specific result. When you need to lighten hair, you can easily explain to the client why natural pigments must be considered by showing what happens when you take a red crayon and color over black.

CORKSCREW CURLS

The "old" definition was for permed or roller set curls that were spiralled around a rod or roller, creating a Shirley Temple look. In braiding, the Corkscrew curl is similar to a Senegalese twist. Thread (visible or invisible) is used to create and secure the corkscrew effect.

CORNROWS

Inverted or underhand three-strand braids. They're created by alternately crossing the two outer strands underneath the center strand. They can be on the scalp or off the scalp. In the West Indies, they're called *canerows*.

CORTEX

The second layer of hair that is most affected by chemical services. It contains fibers of hard keratin, which make up polypeptide chains, linked by bonds. The peptide bonds are the strongest chemical bonds; cross-bonds, which are broken and reformed during perming and relaxing, are either sulfur (chemical bonds) or hydrogen (physical). Sulfur and hydrogen bonds hold the polypeptide bonds in position. Color molecules and melanosomes are also found in the cortex. This little bit of chemistry can be used to explain to clients why you are refusing a chemical service. Each time hair is permed or relaxed, a few cross-bonds do not reform. That's bad enough, but after a while hair gets so weak that the peptide bonds that cross-bonds hold in place can be affected. If that happens, hair is severely damaged, and only cutting it off will save it.

CURL CONFIGURATION

This refers to the shape of the curl. (Also called *curl speed, curl pattern*.) Curl can be extremely tight and coiled, medium or moderately curly, *S*-shaped, loosely *S*-shaped, slightly waved or straight. There are many variations in between. The curl configuration is most important when analyzing hair to perform chemical services. While "excessively curly" has often been used to describe classic African hair, this raises the question: excessive compared to what? The implication is that there is a normal and abnormal way for hair to curl. The best approach is to look at an *S*-shape as being the midpoint on a scale. Hair at one end of the scale is extremely straight; hair at the other end of the scale is extremely curly.

CURLY PERM, OR A CURL

(Also called *curl reformation*.) Once, perming was thought of as adding curl. Today perming solution is being used to straighten hair; many African Americans call a relaxing service a perm because the result is permanent. Since clients think in terms of end results, discuss perms in those terms. "Do you want your hair straight or curly?" The terms *curly perm* or *curl* make the end result clear. Then consider how it is done—by using a one or a two-step technique. When permanent wave solution is used to straighten hair in a single step, it's usually referred to as a *reverse perm*, a *straight perm*. Sometimes a curly perm is referred to by a product name, such as Jheri Curl. Thinking of perms as being done in one or two steps simplifies the processes in your mind.

CUTICLE

The first, or outermost, layer of hair. What matters to you most is how porous or compact the cuticle is, and this can easily be observed.

DEMI-PERMANENT COLOR

A new category of color, also called no lift/no ammonia; no peroxide; long-lasting, semi-permanent; deposit only. Demi-permanent colors have the gentleness of semi-permanent color, but last longer than traditional semi-permanent colors due to their unique chemistry. Most of them use a developer, and no matter what the developer or "activator" is called, it almost always contains some hydrogen peroxide. What interests clients most is the marketing aspect. Along with the "natural" movement came an aversion to ammonia and peroxide. Therefore, these colors are most easily described to clients by what they don't contain and the end result, which is the fact that they last longer than semi-permanent colors.

DENSITY

The abundance (or sparseness) of hair, or the number of single strands of hair per square inch. To clients, this describes whether their hair is thick or thin. Sometimes clients describe fine hair as being thin, but to hairdressers, fine describes the diameter of the individual strand. The difference is worth explaining to a client, because it can result in a positive: "Your hair is fine but you have lots of it." (Good news!)

DEVELOPER

A developer is an oxidizing agent, usually a hydrogen peroxide solution, which is mixed with a haircolor product to supply the necessary oxygen to create a desired chemical reaction. Once developers were described as being mixed with aniline derivative tints only, but in today's creative techniques, developers are sometimes mixed with demi- and semi-permanent colors and even with color-enhancing shampoos. For chemical purposes, keep in mind that developers almost always change or break down melanin pigments.

DOUBLE PROCESS

Double processing is coloring in two steps. First the hair is lightened, then tone is added back. (Also called two-step tinting.) Clients tend to use the word *bleaching* for a double-process color, because they are unaware that two steps are required for other processes as well as for creating pale blondes. It is increasingly important to explain the process, because brunettes are unaware of what it takes to turn very dark brown into true red. Also, double-process color services cannot be performed on relaxed hair or hair that has had a two-step perm. Even double processing hair that has been permed in a single step is risky; never attempt it without taking a test curl. It should be simple to explain that more than one aggressive chemical service can result in over-processing and why. When all else fails, clients understand what "fried" means.

DRABBER

A drabber is a haircoloring product that contains either blue or ash tones and no reds or golds. A drabber is used to offset brassiness in hair.

ETHNIC

Market researchers who want to track product sales by market segment often use the word *ethnic*. Although in some areas it can mean Irish or Italian, it has come to represent exclusion to many because the clear implication is "not white." There's no reason not to call people what they are; your greater concern is the client's hair type. Hair doesn't know whose head it's on.

EXTENSIONS

Extensions are hair additions, usually added to extend length.

FADE

A fade is a technique for cutting in which hair is clipper cut extremely close to the head at the bottom and left longer at the top. The two areas slowly fade into one another, with no obvious lines or steps. Variations describe the finished effect: the close fade, the high-top fade, the ramp. As you'll note, the name usually puts the focus on the shape of the longer top hair.

FADE-OFF

Permanent color is not totally permanent. As time goes by, some fade-off occurs and underlying pigment, which was affected by developer, shows through. That's how you get brass.

FILLERS

Fillers, which are made up of a jelly-like substance, protein, keratin and certified color, are named for their action, or end result. They have similar chemical properties as hair; therefore they fill in porosity and even it out. They can also be used to deposit a base prior to tinting. One of their best uses is with reds, which tend to fade easily, especially at the ends of the hair shaft.

FOLLICLE

The folllicle is the pocket-like structure that encases the hair's root, below the scalp.

FREEFORM

A technique for applying haircolor that follows no set pattern. Color is painted on with brushes or even applied by hand.

GODDESS BRAIDS

These are large inverted braids created along a wide parting, as opposed to within an individual section. They are almost always created with a long free end so they can be styled into an updo.

HAIR ADDITIONS

Hair (human or synthetic) that's added to the head in any temporary form, including the attachment of wefts, braids or hair integration systems are called hair additions. Additions can be used to add volume, length, density, color and texture. Implants and plugs aren't additions because they are theoretically permanent; wigs aren't called additions because they sit on the head—they are not integrated into the existing hair. This blanket term is useful for headlines in promotions or on window signs, followed by specific techniques that clients will want.

HAIR REPLACEMENT

Hair replacement refers to any number of methods for replacing hair, including using wigs, toupees, integration systems or hair additions. With the "graying of America," or seventy million aging baby boomers, hair replacement skills will be in increased demand.

HBA

Health and beauty aids are known by this acronym. This catch-all term is used by market researchers and includes items as diverse as shampoo and deodorant.

INTERLOCK

Interlock is a system of periodically and systematically adding multiple strands of hair to the center of a three-strand braid or incorporating synthetic hair into a braid to strengthen it. Regionally techniques vary widely, and many braiders have created specific names for their own systems. Clients like it because of the end result: stronger, longer-lasting braids that can even be created when the client's natural hair is sparse or fine. Interlocking with synthetic fiber can help somewhat slippery straight hair hold a braid.

INTERNATIONAL BRAIDERS NETWORK (IBN)

The IBN was founded in 1992, to further the cause of braiding and promote education in braiding. It now holds its own show and offers classes; it is active in promoting legislation beneficial to braiders, who do not want or need complete fledged cosmetology licenses.

KERATIN

Keratin is the hard protein of which hair is comprised.

LIGHTENING

Removing natural pigment or artificial color from hair is lightening. (Also called decolorizing by professionals, bleaching by clients.) All permanent tints lighten hair prior to depositing color. Lightening products include oil, cream and powder lighteners. For the most part, clients think of lightening in terms of final results, and take "lighter" quite literally. Describe any final result in terms of brightness, richness, tone, depth, shine and so forth.

LIN

Lin is a hair fiber made from an African plant, which is used to create larger braids, such as Casamas. Lin looks and feels incredibly natural but cannot be shampooed. It can be found through beauty supply houses that serve the African-American market and African import companies.

LOCKTICIAN

A locktician specializes in cultivating hair locks.

MARKETING

Marketing was once defined as a total plan that addressed the famous four "*Ps*": product, price, place and promotion. A more modern interpretation was coined by Linda LoRe, the president of Giorgio, Beverly Hills. It replaces the "*Ps*" with the four "*Cs*": customer, cost, convenience and communication. Blend all these for business success.

MEDULLA

The innermost layer of hair is the medulla, which is made up of a loose arrangement of cells. Its function is uncertain; it can be destroyed or absent in very fine hair.

MELANOSOMES

Located in the cortex, these house melanin, which is responsible for hair color.

NATURAL HAIRSTYLING AND NATURAL HAIRSTYLISTS

Hairstyling and hair care without the use of chemicals or thermal tools is called natural hairstyling. Natural hairstylists go beyond braiding and styling, specializing in natural approaches to total hair care. New York State currently has a separate license for natural hairstylists; Washington D.C. is developing the curriculum for one. Some states have separate licenses for braiders, but these fall short of natural hairstyling licenses. If you interpret the law literally, braiders cannot shampoo hair, because shampoo is a chemical; natural hairstylists can shampoo hair. A related term is *cultural hairstylist*. They emphasize cultural styles and the spirituality and pride in their creation. Many of the techniques used by these professionals were passed down by word of mouth.

OVERBRAID

Overbraid is a "regular" braid or a three-strand braid that is created by alternately crossing outside strands over the center strand.

PAPILLA

The cone-shaped elevation at the very bottom of the follicle is the papilla. It fits into the bulb and provides the blood supply and nourishment to the hair.

PATCH TEST

A test performed on the skin to predict an allergic reaction prior to a chemical service. In reality, salons rarely perform it, but in an increasingly litigious society, it is highly recommended.

PERMANENT WAVE

(See curly perm.) Traditionally, a permanent wave is curl created by using a thioglycolic lotion and wrapping the hair on rods. In the two-step perm, the hair is straightened first, using a reducing cream; then it is permed using a thio-based lotion or cream, or a curl booster.

PERMANENT HAIRCOLOR

Oxidative color or an oxidative tint is permanent. Clients think it lasts forever; in reality it fades in various degrees, depending on the product line. With fade-off appears brass.

pH

Literally, pH stands for potential hydrogen. The pH scale measures the degree of acidity or alkalinity on a scale of 0 to 14. 1 is very acid; 14 is highly alkaline; 7 is neutral. Hair is balanced between 4.5 and 5.5. Thio relaxers and cold-wave solutions have a pH range of 9.4 to 9.6; sodium hydroxide relaxers have a pH of 10 to 14. The pH of lighteners is about 10; semi-permanent haircolor is alkaline; neutralizers are always acid. When talking to clients, the primary focus should be the hair's natural pH and how you will return it to that balanced state.

PIGGYBACK WRAP

A wrap used during permanent waving in which two or more rods are wrapped on a single strand of hair is called a piggypack.

PRESSING

A press is a method of straightening very curly hair or temporarily changing its texture by pressing it with a hot comb or pressing iron, while using a light pressing oil. Soft pressing uses 250 degrees of heat. Hard pressing is performed at a temperature of 300 to 350 degrees. In the hard press, the top of a section is pressed twice; then the underside is pressed. The technique provides an alternative to chemical straightening.

PROJECTION ANGLE

The projection angle is the angle at which hair is held out from the head while cutting. Also called elevation.

RASTAFARIAN LOCKS

Locks are formed when hair is allowed to go its own way and reflect the effects of elements such as sun, water and sand. They are matted in appearance; any type of hair can mat in this manner if left unattended. Rastafarian locks have religious significance to many and should not be referred to as *dreads* or *Dreadlocks*, which is a negative connotation that reflects the reaction of early Europeans when they first viewed the style.

REFORMATION

Reformation is another word for perming or chemical reformation. Simplify life and stick to *perming*.

RELAXER

A chemical applied to curly hair in order to straighten it is a relaxer. It is still called a chemical blow-out by some clients and stylists. When hair is relaxed, the curl pattern is usually reduced by 80 to 90 percent.

RESTRUCTURING

Taking hair that has been chemically relaxed with a sodium hydroxide product and applying another chemical to add curl is called restructuring. While some manufacturers claim that their products permit this safely, avoid this procedure. Hair breakage is certain. A better solution is to straighten the hair with a thio-based product, which will allow you to chemically curl it later if the client changes his or her mind.

ROOT

The root is the hair below the scalp. Clients call the hair right at the scalp the roots, which is why you'll hear them ask for a "root" press or say their roots are showing. This doesn't really present any communication problem, but, if you prefer, you can try to get them in the habit of thinking of this hair as the new growth or regrowth when referring to chemically treated hair.

SEMI-PERMANENT HAIRCOLOR

Color that is formulated to last from four to six weeks is semi-permanent. Semi-permanent colors are oxidizing (or aniline derivative) tints, but have much larger molecules than permanent tints do. They do not require the use of a developer or hydrogen peroxide, but some colorists add a small amount of low-volume developer for effect. Alkaline shampoos open the cuticle, allowing these molecules to pass out; therefore, a pH balanced shampoo or color-enhancing shampoo will extend the life of semi-permanent color.

SENEGALESE TWISTS

Braids are created by twisting two strands of hair from an individual section. The hair is rolled, then intertwined.

SHAFT

The shaft is the long, slender part of the hair that we see because it's above the scalp.

SODIUM HYDROXIDE

Sodium hydroxide is an ingredient in relaxer that is extremely alkaline. Lay persons think of it as the lye in the product. A sodium hydroxide product is not compatible with a thio-based product.

STRAIGHTENER

This is another term for a relaxer. Straightening can also be temporary when thermal tools are used. If a client wants the hair straightened, clarify the technique—chemical or thermal.

STRAIGHT PERM

A term that really refers to the final result. Permanent wave solution is used to straighten hair in one of several techniques. The hair can be wrapped around the head, placed on long strips prior to application of the solution, or dangled straight down while the product is repeatedly combed through the hair.

STRAND TEST

A precaution taken when performing chemical services. A strand of hair (usually one at the nape and underneath others, so it cannot be seen if the test fails) is treated with the chosen chemical to determine a number of factors, such as reaction, timing, product strength and feasibility of the service. It's your insurance against losing your insurance, so to speak. A strand test should always be performed when hair is receiving more than one chemical service; when bleaching or lightening hair that is very porous or has a very compact cuticle; when hair is fragile, porous or contains henna or metallic salts; when you're uncertain of results. Good sense dictates that a strand test should be performed with every first-time client, or any time the hair or the chemical being used changes. It will not frighten clients if presented as a way to see if they like the results.

TEMPORARY HAIRCOLOR

Temporary haircolor only coats the cuticle and washes out after a single shampoo.

TENSILE STRENGTH

Tensile strength refers to how much pull or pressure a strand of hair can take before it breaks.

TEXTURE

Texture is the diameter of a hair strand or feel of it, which classifies it as coarse, medium or fine.

TEXTURIZE

Texturizing is done by applying a relaxer to reduce the curl pattern by a specific percentage or degree. Generally the goal is to retain wave or curl and reduce the curl pattern by a far lesser degree than relaxing does. Any type of hair that is curly can be texturized.

TOUCH-UP

Application of a haircolor product, relaxing product or permanent wave solution to new growth only is a touch-up. The more aggressive the chemical, the greater care you must take not to overlap the product onto previously treated hair.

TRACKS

A parting or on-the-scalp braid that establishes the placement pattern of hair additions, which will be attached to the tracks.

UNDERBRAID

An underbraid is a three-strand braid that is created by crossing outside strands alternately under the center strand. Another name for this is inverted braid. Use it as a noun (the braid) or a verb (the act).

UNDERLYING PIGMENT

The color molecules in the cortex are the underlying pigment, which become diffused when they react with hydrogen peroxide. Very dark hair has red underlying pigment, which must be kept in mind when attempting to color it without seeing brass.

WEAVING

Weaving is a technique for creating tracks that incorporates the use of thread. The resulting tracks are stronger and more secure. In general language, clients refer to adding hair additions as "hair weaving" and refer to additions as "a weave."

WEFTS

Wefts are strands of human or synthetic hair that have been sewn along a single edge to create a long line of hair. Wefts can be cut to any width desired and attached to tracks or bonded to the hair.

ZERO PROJECTION

You are using zero projection when you hold the hair as close to the head as possible when you cut; not elevating it at all.

THE MOST COMMON AREAS OF MISCOMMUNICATION

Part of having a professional, client-centered vocabulary is putting it to use when it counts the most. What follows are the most common areas of miscommunication in the salons.

LAYERS

Clients have a range of ideas about what layers are, but thanks to misunderstanding, most are a bit afraid of them. "Why don't we layer your hair?" conjures up images of too-short, chopped-up hair for many, and Farrah Fawcett "wings" for others. The best way to introduce layers is to ask the client if she likes her hair all one length and to ask what her chief complaints are about her hair. Usually what's disliked is lack of movement or volume. Then explain that layers can be very long, subtle and sprinkled throughout the head. Name movie stars, models and singers who have light layers or show the client photos. While many clients are afraid of cutting layers for the first time, if you start with subtle ones, they'll keep asking for them, since they add mobility to most any cut.

TONE

Clients have no idea that, to colorists, level means degree of lightness and darkness, and tone means warm or cool. They think tone means red and rarely stop to think that red can be warm or cool. Rarely do clients ask for a cool or ash color. They communicate with phrases like "Not a bright red, a darker red," "I want a warm brown," and "That color washes me out." The simplest thing any colorist could do is keep a "look book" that contains photos, which are separated by level, and displays warm and cool shades next to each other so clients can see the difference. You don't have to teach them what "level" means, talk about black, brunette, red and blonde, light or dark and then show samples of tone and recommend the appropriate one for the client's skin tone.

BRASS

Most clients mistake red for brass and complain that after a while their hair looks red. Blondes think of brass as harsh gold or even mistake a green cast for brass. Question the client closely to determine exactly what he or she doesn't want to see, and educate yourself thoroughly about contributing and underlying pigment, color formulation and corrective procedures.

PERM

In case you skipped the previous glossary, many African-American clients ask for a perm when they want a relaxing service. Always clarify by asking the client if she means a straightener or a curl. To many other clients, a perm means lots of curl. Always use an adjective to describe your perm when you suggest it—an adjective that takes the emphasis off curl unless that's what the client wants. Suggest body perms and soft waves, or describe the final effect. "You'll get lift just near the scalp."

TRIM

This is a major client complaint. To a client, a trim is a quarter to half an inch; when it comes to most hairdressers, at least an inch hits the floor. This may well be the number one cause of clients never returning. Show the client how much you're going to remove before you do it; show her the first snippet if she's a stickler. Then do what you said you were going to do. If the hair is damaged and more should be removed, explain this, but if the client insists, you can't hurt hair more by complying, so you'd may as well. It's not like proceeding with a chemical service that you know isn't appropriate and that could end in a lawsuit if major breakage occurs.

WHEN THE PRICE DOES NOT INCLUDE STYLING

An increasing number of salons are charging separately for styling. Clients should always be informed of this when they book an appointment. The best way is to ask if they'll need someone to style their hair or if they'll be styling their own. Go on to let them know you provide tools for this. If a client was not told about this when she booked and was not prepared to style her own hair, its best to do it free of charge for one time.

WHY YOU REFUSE TO PERFORM A SERVICE

If you know a chemical service requested will damage hair or isn't right for the client, take the time to explain why. Some salons guarantee their work only if the client follows the salon's recommendations for both services and retail. If the client insists or threatens to go elsewhere, let someone else do the damage. Politely but firmly refuse, reiterating your concern for the client's hair. Then offer to be available for corrective hair care if the client does go elsewhere.

WHY SALON PRODUCTS COST MORE

Face it, clients can get shampoos at the supermarket for a couple of dollars. Become informed about ingredients and their effect on hair to be able to compare supermarket shampoos with yours; ask your manufacturer or distributor for assistance. Haircolor clients are the easiest to talk to, because you can explain how much they just spent for haircolor that shampoos can strip. Recommend the salon's color-enhancing or color-protecting product. Chemical service clients need to maintain what they just paid for and have special hair-moisture needs. If the client isn't convinced, give out samples. If your salon carries more than one product line with different price points, you'll be able to suggest alternatives that suit the client's budget.

WHY THE CLIENT CAN'T REPRODUCE THE STYLE SHE LEFT THE SALON WEARING

Clients don't expect to be hairdressers, but they do expect to be able to style your new cut; if they can't, they think the cut is bad. Always give the client tips as you finish the hair. Offer free styling lessons during the evening or down time and invite all your clients, also inviting them to bring friends. It's a great way to stand out from other stylists and to get new clients.

WHY YOU'RE RUNNING LATE

No matter what you communicate, forget trying to explain why you're running late or offering excuses. A well-trained receptionist should inform the client and immediately offer her some sort of complimentary service while she's waiting, if it will be unreasonably long. A manicure, deep-conditioning treatment, five-minute color refresher or a mini facial are excellent options that help the salon build business in other areas.

WHY YOU CHARGE MORE FOR MEN, WOMEN, BLACK HAIR, LONG HAIR, ETC.

One of the reasons salons started charging separately for styling was in response to lawsuits being brought for charging less for men's cuts than women's. Much of women's appointment time was being spent on styling. If you still want to make more on complex women's styles, set a men's, women's and long-hair price. The latter applies to either sex.

Long or very dense hair takes much longer to highlight or perm than super-short hair. Solutions include charging by the rod or foil (which allows you to offer quick spot perms and trial highlights at reasonable cost) or to set two or three price ranges for these chemical services, based on short hair, medium-length hair and long hair. (If the client quibbles about medium versus long, vote with the client.)

A number of salons have been sued recently for charging more for "black hair." In every case documented, the salon told the client it was "harder to do." If you are well-trained and well-educated in working with all types of hair, no hair is harder to do than any other, and you should never charge clients a higher price based on race.

INDEX

References in bold represent illustrations.

I

V

Velcro rollers, 124
Virgin hair
    gray coverage for, 229-30
    relaxer service, 147-49, **148-49**
    two-step perm, 163-66

W

Walker, Madame C.J., 29-30
Washington, Sarah Spencer, 30-31
Wavy hair, styling, 244-45
Weaving, 82, 182-84, 318
Wedding styles, 246
    braids, 251-53
    headpieces, 248
    mid-length, layered cuts, **249-50**, 249-51
    pre-wedding time line, 247-48
Wedge, 80, **80**, 107-9, **108-9**
Wefts, 193-94, 319
Wet-on-wet technique, 222-23

Wig
    cutting, 82-83, **83**, 272
    home care of, 272-73
Women
    advanced cuts for, 88-99
    cost for styling, 321-22
    hair loss solutions for, 265-71
Wrapping, **130-31**, 130-31, 240
Wrapping techniques (perms)
    alternating wraps, 161-62
    bricklaying, 160-61, 308
    piggyback, 161, 315
    for short hair, 163
    stack wrapping, 162

Z

Zero projection, 319
Z-shaped lines, 245-46

LIBRARY
RUGBY COLLEGE

NOTES

LIBRARY
RUGBY COLLEGE

Style.
Savvy.
Solutions.

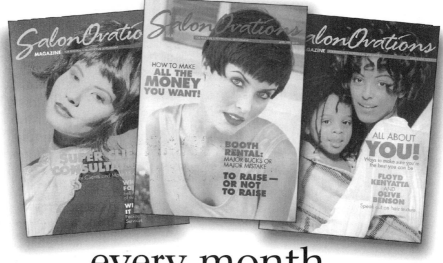

every month.
SalonOvations

SalonOvations is a professional and personal magazine designed with you in mind. Each issue delivers great features on personal growth and on-target stories about the beauty business. Get helpful hints from industry pros on starting your own salon business and how to satisfy your clients. Plus, you'll get pages of colorful photos of the latest trends in haircutting, styling and coloring.

All this at a great price of 12 **15** issues for only $19.95 a year! **3 FREE issues** - Save over 40% (price subject to change)

YES! Send me **3 FREE** issues of *SalonOvations Magazine* plus 12 issues at the special low rate of $19.95! That's a total of 15 issues for the price of 12! – A $33.75 value – **Save over 40%**

Name _____

Signature _____
(order cannot be processed without a signature)

Title _____

Salon or School Name _____

Your Mailing Address _____

City/State/Zip _____

Phone _____

❏ Here's my check or money order for $19.95 ❏ MasterCard ❏ VISA

Card# _____ Exp Date _____

Job Title: ❏ Student ❏ Hair Colorist ❏ Esthetician ❏ Salon Owner ❏ Teacher/Educator
❏ Hair Stylist ❏ Barber ❏ Nail Technician ❏ Salon Mgr. ❏ Mfr's Rep ❏ Other_____

Type of Business: ❏ School ❏ Full Svc. Salon ❏ Skin Care Salon ❏ Beauty Supply Dist.
❏ Beauty Salon ❏ Nail Salon ❏ Resort or Spa ❏ Manufacturer ❏ Other_____

Clip and mail to: *SalonOvations* Subscriptions, PO Box 10520, Riverton, NJ 08706-8520   code 95013